ALZHEIMER'S DISEASE

A RELENTLESS MULTI-DIMENSIONAL ILLNESS

(with a multi-pronged strategy, fighting against a growing epidemic)

Dr. Richard Ng, D.O.

ISBN 978-1-956696-63-9 (paperback)
ISBN 978-1-956696-64-6 (hardcover)
ISBN 978-1-956696-65-3 (digital)

Rushmore Press LLC
1 800 460 9188
www.rushmorepress.com

Printed in the United States of America

MISSION STATEMENTS

The mission for writing this book is at least three-fold:

1. To inform the public and readers for better understanding of the unpredictable and devastating nature of Alzheimer's disease, to dispel any of its myths, and to encourage and bolster awareness of the mitigating and aggravating factors in the development of this terrible illness.
2. To lend supports, both mentally and spiritually, to the loving, grieving and steadfast caregivers on their long, grueling journey with their silently suffering loved ones.
3. To help patients inflicted with this cruel, protracted and devastating disease to have some quality of life and dignity with as much as independence and inter-dependence in their struggles. Along with continuing research and social understanding, we can slow and halt the progression of the disease and hopefully reverse its course.

AUTHOR'S NOTES

The information presented in this book is based on medical education and training, personal experiences and observation, extensive research and review of many medical publications on the subject matter.

Sensible and judicious approach by the readers is recommended. The adoption of certain information in this book should be done under the professional supervision and with the advice of the attending physicians.

With so many possible contributing factors to the development of Alzheimer's Disease, the concept of individualized therapeutic approach will serve the patients best with this multi-dimensional and multi-causal chronic illness.

ABOUT THE AUTHOR

A naturalized U.S. citizen originally from China, Dr. Richard Ng, D.O. received his medical degree from Midwestern University the Chicago College of Osteopathic Medicine. The 19-month incarceration at the Federal Medical Center in Rochester, Minnesota, was very tormenting in the beginning. However, the experience of this confinement was both informative and transformative for me. It has transformed my life with a new, perspective of life, and has helped me to embrace the meaning of purpose of our existence.

The Federal Medical Center, a low-security facility, has a general hospital and a mental health building in addition to the inmate quarters. I had the trusted opportunity to work as an inmate-companion, doing fall watch at the hospital for the sick fellow inmates with various illnesses including Alzheimer's Disease and other forms of dementia. As an inmate companion, I also worked in the unit at the mental health center for suicide watch after completion of classes for suicide watch taught by psychologists and psychiatrists.

The incarceration at the Federal Medical Center, which is about one mile from the Mayo Clinic and its medical school, provided me with much focused time and available resources to continue my research and study about Alzheimer's Disease. It is such a scourge, and it is the most terrible, devastating thing that can befall anyone who think!

How many more minds Alzheimer's Disease is going to dismantle and destroy before we can stop it on its track? I know we can do it so that we can cherish our memories and dreams, appreciate our identities, and pass on our wisdom and meaningful legacies with a graceful finale. This is the existential difference between the human beings and other animal species!

ACKNOWLEDGEMENT

With much love to my four children, David, Thomas, Kevin and Sarah, the precious gifts from God for Whom I am forever grateful. I am also thankful to my wife, Mary Kathleen Balgemann Ng, who has done a wonderful job in raising them!

Life is eternal, and Love is immortal; and death is only a horizon; and a horizon is nothing save the limit of our sight.

By Rossiter Worthington Raymond
(1840 – 1918)

PREMISE

It is my belief that Alzheimer's Disease, a neuro-degenerative process, is caused by the neurotoxic micro-environment generated by oxidative stress in the brain. Oxidative stress is the most important underlying pathogenesis in the development of Alzheimer's Disease.

Transmission between neurons and nerves is a matter of chemistry --- the foundation on which neuroscience is built. Excessive amounts of free radicals, the toxic molecules either coming from sources outside the body or inside the body, are associated with the development of Alzheimer's Disease and other illnesses such as cancers, atherosclerosis, stroke and heart disease. The elevated levels of free radicals can overwhelm the protective mechanism of the body, tilting the body's equilibrium and resulting in damages to the DNA, proteins and lipid membranes, the brain in particular.

We should be able to prevent degenerative diseases if oxidative stress can be prevented. Realistically, we know that elimination of oxidative stress is not possible; but we must look for other factors that can alleviate and reduce its levels and protect us against oxidative stress. Many research studies have shown that oxidative stress alone is sufficient to cause dementia in seniors who have no known risk factors. It is undeniable that Alzheimer's Disease is associated with aging and aging is a function of oxidative stress. Antioxidants, either internal (endogenous) or external (exogenous or supplemental), are not a panacea for Alzheimer's Disease and other age-related illnesses; they are important parts of the solution.

We should not focus on the genes that increase our susceptibility to dementia, and in so doing, we may have the chance not only to prevent dementia, but at the same time to decrease other age-related diseases. Just to increase our life span is not enough, we must match it with health span.

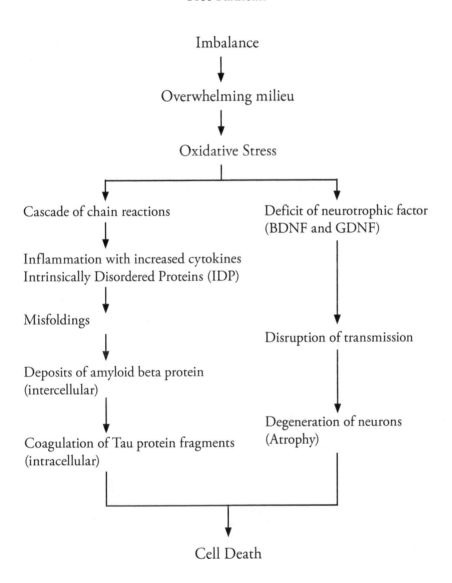

CONTENTS

INTRODUCTION

According to some social studies, when one gets into adulthood or older, the three illnesses people seem to fear most are cancer, heart disease and Alzheimer's Disease. Today, Alzheimer's Disease probably has surpassed cancer and heart disease in America, and likely the most feared disease in the Western world.

At the present time, there are about 4.8 million people diagnosed and suffering from the disease in the U.S. Advances in medical sciences have helped to fight and conquer many human diseases such as pneumonia, malaria the common childhood diseases and AIDS, but ironically allowing people to live long enough to develop the most heart-breaking and relentless illness of Alzheimer's.

Admittedly, we are still struggling with quite a few chronic diseases including the three already mentioned, and the irony is the older one becomes, the higher the risk for those terrible chronic diseases, Alzheimer's in particular. Alzheimer's Disease is not an actual consequence of aging or a normal part of aging, it is essentially a disease of older people, the sporadic, late-onset form. Unfortunately, Alzheimer's is the most common type of dementia.

The gradual loss of memory with worsening symptoms of dementia as the illness progresses is very frightening for most, if not all of us. Practically, the afflicted individuals are putting their identities on hold, losing the frame of references and their internal systems of "check and balance". It is a tragic disconnect from life!

Medical researchers, who have been tirelessly and fastidiously trying and scrambling to develop effective treatments for Alzheimer's

1

Disease for more than three decades, have so far come away essentially empty-handed. No drug has been shown to stop, reverse or even slow the advance of this dementing illness.

Some experts think that certain infections may be the cause of Alzheimer's and suggest that anti-microbial or ant-viral drugs might have possible therapeutic value. But, the possibility of the role of micro-organisms in the development of Alzheimer's Disease is very doubtful. In the absence of drugs that tackle the biological causes of the disease, more and more doctors are turning to a more holistic approach.

The brains of individuals with the diagnosis of Alzheimer's disease at autopsies, though not in all of them, show two cellular hallmarks: aggregates of beta-amyloid plaques outside the neurons, and strings a misfolded tau-protein, known as neuro-fibrillary tangles inside the neurons. Both deposits were first described more than a century ago in 1906 by Dr. Lois Alzheimer in Germany. Both plaques and tangles can be found together; however, they can exist in the absence of other.

According to the beta-amyloid hypothesis, the plaques are thought to trigger a cascade of abnormal processes such as inflammation, MISFOLDING OF PROTEINS LEADING TO THE FORMATION OF TAU TANGLES, SYNAPTIC dysfunction, breakdown and eventual death of neurons, thus loss of memory and cognitive ability. It is understandable that beta-amyloid has become an obvious therapeutic target.

Nevertheless, the beta-amyloid plaques are also found in the brains of many elderly people with intact memory and cognitive functions. Studies based on post-mortem examinations revealed that about half of the patients who were clinically diagnosed with Alzheimer's Disease did not have the signature pathological changes in the brains, i.e. plaques and tangles were absent.

In fact, the appearance of beta-amyloid plaques is a normal physiological process that occurs even in healthy people, and the body under normal circumstances can clear away the beta-amyloid proteins. In Alzheimer's patients, these proteins are not being broken down and removed, probably due to abnormally accelerated production of the beta-amyloid peptides. Instead, they stick together to become large, insoluble deposits compromising neuronal functions. Neuroscientific research has shown that the higher the levels of insulin in the blood stream, the more beta-amyloid protein will build up, and thus more likely to form plaques. It is no wonder that diabetes mellitus is a risk factor for the development of Alzheimer's Disease.

The "Tau" protein is found inside the neurons. In order to function properly, a protein must have a 3-dimensional shape, a specific conformation. Folding is a process by which the amino acids that make up the protein twist or fold themselves into a specific conformation. When there is a molecular defect, the "Tau" proteins misfold, resulting in abnormal, toxic clumps called neurofibrillary tangles; coupled with the beta-amyloid plaques, they eventually lead to cell death and progression of the disease.

Reflectively, some of the symptoms such as forgetfulness, confusion, difficulties in organizing the daily activities and communicating with others are not just from stresses or the normal wear and tear in the aging process. It has become clearer and clearer with a plethora of findings that there are many other contributing factors involved in the development of Alzheimer's Disease besides the genes or the plaques and tangles spreading across the brain.

Dr. Dale Bredesen, a professor of Neurology at the UCLA states that based on 30 years of research, "Alzheimer's disease is triggered by a broad range of factors that upset the body's natural process of cell turnover and renewal". He believes that "while these contributors by themselves are not enough to tip the brain into a downward spiral, taken together they have a cumulative effect, resulting in the destruction of neurons and crucial signaling connections between brain cells".

Normally, synapse-forming and synapse-destroying activities are in a dynamic equilibrium as seen in other systems of the body. Alzheimer's disease is a chronic, devastating illness, afflicting up to at least 75% of Americans 85 years of age, based on current available data. Nevertheless, aging may be inevitable, but we have found promising clues and strategies about how to avoid it, slow it down, even reverse it, or how to deal with it in a hopeful, dignified manner.

The human brain, unlike other organs in the body, is very unique. We think of it as who we are because it contains and signifies our identity. It is full of meanings of life --- personal, emotional and spiritual. Graceful aging is certainly possible with many cognitive functions resistant to aging such as wisdom, creativity, the rules of language and reasoning. Lamentably, Alzheimer's disease insidiously and gradually wipes them out.

In general, there is a pessimistic outlook with defeatism when the diagnosis of Alzheimer's disease is delivered and revealed to the patients and their loved ones. I want you to know that Alzheimer's disease is a slow but treatable brain disorder with a considerably large window of opportunity for treatment, especially during the early stages. The dietary and lifestyle factors can have significant, positive impact on the disease process, and these mitigating, neuroprotective factors are entirely within our control! Undoubtedly, the best and earliest intervention of all will be prevention.

In recent years, neuro-scientific studies have shown that the somato-sensory cortex is continuously remodeled throughout life, and plasticity is a general feature of the entire cortex. These studies have demonstrated that the circuits in the cortex can undergo re-organization in response to experience. This cortical plasticity explains why practice makes perfect.

We lose thousands of neurons every day throughout the adult life, resulting in progressive decrease of the gray matter volume, as much as 20% over the life time. Despite death of neurons and shrinkage of brain, most of us do retain our important memories, core personality traits and cognitive abilities under normal circumstances. Neuro-scientists refer to systems that can absorb significant amount of change and damage without dramatic effects on performance as exhibiting 'graceful degradation'. This, paradoxically, is what we should be striving to achieve, especially for individuals suffering from Alzheimer's disease in its early stages.

SIGNS AND SYMPTOMS OF ALZHEIMER'S DISEASE

Alzheimer's disease, a neuro-degenerative disorder of the brain, is so devastating and heart-rending that, unless you have come across people suffering from it, you cannot appreciate the extent of the devastation and loss.

Measurable and subjective signs and symptoms usually appear many years before a diagnosis of Alzheimer's disease is made. They are subtle, but fairly obvious at times; family and friends, without being attentive and suspecting, often disregard those signs and symptoms as parts of getting old. The diagnosis can be missed even by someone who may have some medical training. In fact, misdiagnoses of patients with the disease are not uncommon, especially in the early stages of the illness. Early indicators are imperceptible to the individuals experiencing them, regardless of educational levels.

One of the most common signs of Alzheimer's disease in the early stage is forgetting recently learned information. Others include forgetting important dates or events, asking for the same questions again and again, and needing family members for things they used to handle on their own. The patients have difficulty remembering birthdays, names of people and objects which are familiar. For example, a grandfather who suddenly starts calling his grandchildren by the wrong names. They may repeatedly make the same request or tell the same story over and over because they simply cannot remember what they did or what happened just minutes before.

It is heart-breaking and sad for family to witness the progressive loss of patient's memory, both short-term and long-term, and orientation in time and place. Patient is unable to tell you the season or the month of the year, the day of the week or the time of the day.

Once the diagnosis is confirmed, family and caregivers and close friends are struggling with acceptance and denial, as in a grieving process, and the uncertainty of this impending calamity. The signs and symptoms exhibited by the patients are often variable and unpredictable and their presentations are determined by specific regions involved and the extent of damage in the brain, and the stages of the disease process. The patient may be able to remember things from long time ago, but not from yesterday; the Alzheimer's sufferers will be able to do some things but not others.

It can be very challenging for the patient to develop and follow a plan, or to solve simple problems such as following a recipe or keeping track of monthly bills at home. They may have difficulty concentrating and take a much longer time to do things than they did before. THIS DIFFICULTY IN COMPLETING FAMILIAR TASKS is perceptible, such as having trouble driving to a familiar location because of the loss of ability to reconstruct a route, or remembering the rules of a favorite game. They may lose things and not able to retrace their steps to find them; sometimes they can blame others for taking them, becoming argumentative.

Other warning signs of Alzheimer's disease include visual problems and a poor understanding of spatial relationships and visual images. Fox example, they may pass a mirror and think another person in the room. This can also lead to difficulty with balance, judging distance and determining color or contrast. Driving can become problematic and uneasy partly due to disruption of depth perception.

Other problems in the early stages of the illness; the affected individuals may have trouble following or joining a conversation. They may stop in a discussion or in the middle of a conversation and have no clue how to continue. They often have difficulty finding the correct word or vocabulary, or naming a familiar object, e.g. calling a 'watch' a 'hand-clock'. An Alzheimer's patient may have trouble operating familiar equipment and appliance at home: how to use the microwave or washing machine, for example.

You will notice in a family member or someone you care about not being properly groomed, withdrawing from favorite hobbies and games and other social activities. Persons with Alzheimer's may mood and personality changes, becoming confused, fearful, depressed, suspicious or anxious. They get upset easily and can be furious about things without apparent reasons. A laid-back person who is usually slow to anger and cool under pressure can manifest explosive personality all of a sudden, very angry and saying mean things to people it is never done before.

Cognitive abilities are damaged unevenly and at different times; the Alzheimer's patients will be able to do some things but not others. It is possible for the Alzheimer's disease to damage one part of the brain without damaging the other as much. The gradual loss of taste is rather subtle, and the person with Alzheimer's may show it as "loss of appetite" even for the favorite foods.

Some will have trouble telling the difference between the refrigerator and the freezer; for some patients, even preparing a simple meal such as sandwiches for themselves is challenging and difficult. They can get lost just walking to a familiar place nearby they have visited many times. Some cannot even distinguish the family pet from a household item. The affected person can get lost in the building, forgetting where he or she is supposed to be next.

They move and walk slowly, hesitating and stopping. The Alzheimer's patients need to be accompanied everywhere due to fear of falling or stumbling, because they are no longer aware of or understanding the physical perils around them. It is not surprising that the afflicted individual will walk into a swimming pool full of water without realizing the danger of drowning.

Many day-to-day activities of life such as buttoning and unbuttoning the clothes, tying shoe laces, handling kitchen utensil, and opening the doors of kitchen cabinets will become difficult and awkward, even they have performed the same simple activities many times. As a caregiver, you must be patient, compassionate and steadfast, even without any apology from your dementing loved one.

As a caregiver and the driver for your loved one with Alzheimer's disease, you may wonder and feel bewildered in your car waiting for him or her to approach and get into the car. Sometimes, he or she will keep staring at the car with flat affect and oblivion, looking lost and confounded. You need to understand that his or her connection to the physical plane is slipping away. The patient has damaged neurons with faulty connections, like a lose light bulb; sometimes it may work and fail other times. This explains why the person can do something one day and not another day.

Like one of my patients said one time: "I have the lights on in my house, but I am not home".

Because of their fading abilities in expressing, relating and articulating, you will, as caregivers, family members or close friends, find long silences and pauses during conversations. The affected person, while sitting at the dining table eating with family, can lapse into complete silence, taring in the space and absorbed in thought for some time.

As caregiver and a loving spouse, you will never know what the next loss or shock will surface in front of you. One minute, they can be almost their old selves, the next, very different and disconnected. Some of the most disturbing and nerve-wracking symptoms are emotional: the person may show mood swings, experience depression, delusions, withdrawal, paranoia or even aggressive behaviors.

Most patients with Alzheimer's disease can live five to ten years after diagnosis, but some can live as long as 20 years, depending on other factors. In actuality, changes in the brain associated with Alzheimer's start years before any signs of the disease. This time period is referred to as preclinical Alzheimer's disease.

Alzheimer's disease are separated into three stages: early-stage (mild), middle-stage (moderate), and late-stage (severe). Since Alzheimer's disease affects people in different ways, each person may experience symptoms and signs differently while progressing through the stages.

In the early stage of Alzheimer's, the affected individual may live and function independently; he or she may still drive, work and be part of many social activities with some memory lapses. During this early stage of the disease, it is possible for the patients to live well by taking control of their health and wellness.

During the middle stage of the disease, which happens to be the longest stage, the symptoms of dementia are more pronounced with confusion and the person may require a higher level of care. As the need for more intensive care increases in this stage, family members and caregivers may want to consider respite care or an adult day so that the caregivers can have temporary break from caregiving while the person suffering from Alzheimer's continues to receive appropriate care in a safe environment.

In the late stage of Alzheimer's disease, the symptoms are severe with very limited physical abilities such as walking, sitting and even swallowing. Communications are minimal and difficult, with a few or short, simple phrases at best. As the memory and cognitive skills continue to worsen, significant and disturbing personality changes may take place and patients really need extensive care. Dementia becomes more pronounced and less manageable, making independent living essentially impossible and dangerous. They become totally bed-ridden and incontinent. At this time, hospice can be of great benefit to both the caregivers and patient in the final stage of Alzheimer's.

In fact, nobody really knows or can predict how this dementing illness will unfold. It is such an agonizing, cruel process to see how Alzheimer's destroys the mind with physical and mental decline over time. Most of us take for granted the easy transition from sleeping to waking, from one state of consciousness to another. This is not so when the mind is impaired in patients with Alzheimer's disease.

Many of them wake up and do not know what they are going to do or where they are going, and unable to find a purpose. Of course, this is very unsettling, saddening and depressing for the caregiver facing uncertainty every day; I do not doubt that the patient probably feels the same.

Nobody, even the best expert, can figure out what the impaired person understood or intended because the brain is so complex. The best strategy for the caregiver is to remind yourself that a damaged brain is at work, and that it is not something you did or something the impaired person intended.

If you recognize some of the signs and symptoms in a family member or someone you care about, it is important to talk with a healthcare provider. Trust your instinct and 'gut feeling'. Denial is common during the early stages of Alzheimer's disease by the victim, and by the loving family members. Although there is no cure for Alzheimer's disease, you should seek advice from and work with a healthcare professional who can diagnose the condition and recommend the best ways to manage symptoms and provide support. On this long journey of trials and tribulations, pain and suffering, as a caregiver, you are traveling together with your loved one with brain impairments. You will need to pray for wisdom, strength, and equanimity to endure.

One striking thing I want to share with my readers who are taking care of someone with a diagnosis of Alzheimer's disease, or, you are suspecting someone in the family who may have this dementing illness. When my wife survived a major stroke in 2018, her MRIs of the brain confirmed the stroke and the amyloid

Deposition. Her recovery from the stroke was remarkable with physical therapy and rehabilitation, but she seems to have lost her smiles along with some of the signs and symptoms suggestive of Alzheimer's. She does not get excited or take joy in life's simple pleasures such as her favorable meal, funny jokes I tell, or hilarious sitcom on TV. This withdrawal from enjoyed activities, and the inexplicable and profound loss of feeling pleasure can be one of the early signs of Alzheimer's disease and dementia. This lack of or impaired ability to experience pleasure, anhedonia, is discovered by a recent study conducted at the University of Sidney in Australia of patients diagnosed of Fronto-Temporal Dementia (FTD). I think that anhedonia is observed by many caregivers of Alzheimer's patients also, and can be caused by degeneration and deterioration of the brain's pleasure center.

One interesting recent study in France, looking at post-Covid patients four months after the infection, found that 34% of the patients reported memory loss, 28% had trouble concentrating, and 31% had sleep problems.

MEMORIES

Alzheimer's disease is a slow, progressive brain illness, belonging to the class of neuro-degenerative disorders, with memory loss, changes in behavior and personality, and a decline in cognitive abilities. It is a devastating, consumptive and de-moralizing illness; many of the victims end up bed-ridden and completely dependent in the late stages and eventually succumb to infections such as pneumonia and other comorbidities.

The role of memory is very pervasive in our everyday life. There is no one specific part of the brain solely responsible for all memories, though there are certain regions of the brain related to specific memory subsystems. In other words, memory is not a single system that relies on one neuro-anatomical circuit, rather, memory consists of multiple systems that can work independently of one another. Nevertheless, the hippocampus is very important memory region of the limbic system, the oldest area of the brain; it is critical for the ability to learn new information.

Occasionally, some memory slippage is normal as you age, such as misplacing your car keys, forgetting a word, or name of a co-worker, or unable to find your wallet in the house. These small memory lapses are minor problems which can happen to all of us as we get older. This benign condition is called age-related memory loss, and should not be confused with Alzheimer's disease. Some 'senior moments' are part of age-related memory loss and is reversible with the right mental exercises.

Nowadays, there is much anxiety about memory loss associated with Alzheimer's, receiving more and more publicity. Under normal circumstances, the secret of memory is attention, and the secret of attention is motivation. If your attention and/or interest are/is not in the right place and moment when something goes by, you will not remember it no matter how good your memory is.

Some memory problems are treatable when the offending, contributing causes are identified and corrected. The following is a list of condition that can cause poor or sub-optimal memory:

- Anemia
- Dehydration
- Infections
- Sensory losses such as hearing and vision
- Nutritional deficiency such as low blood levels of B12
- Toxic environment due to neurotoxic elements
- Hypothyroidism
- Hypoxia
- Depression
- Anxiety and chronic stresses
- Loneliness and social isolation
- Poly-pharmacy
- Stroke of certain region of the brain
- Tumors of the brain
- Sleep deprivation with fatigue
- Unhealthy lifestyle such as alcohol.
- Use and abuse of illicit drugs

In fact, most of our memory complaints in our daily life stem from the lack of attention; nothing is recorded in our brain in the first place, hence there is nothing to recall. Quite often, we see but do not look, we feel without being aware of it, and hear casually and superficially without listening. After all, by paying attention, you will ensure that all the circuitries in the brain, sensory and intellectual, are open and active. By associating the image and message, you will make a better recording and impression on your memory track.

Perception and memory are intricately entwined. Recognizing a friend, a word or a tune requires not merely linking together different aspects of the perceptual input, but connecting these fragments to the stored memories of faces, words and melodies. So, the interpretation of the information flowing through our senses depends on a body of remembered information, but this information is really nothing more than the memory of past interpretation of previous sensory information. In essence, today's memories are yesterday's perceptual interpretation.

Generally speaking, there are three types of memory in our everyday life:

1. Sensory memory:
   It is the very first, initial kind of memory that enters the brain. It gets your attention for just a split second, enough time for you to sense the environment. For example, the touch of your clothes against the skin, the smell of burning leaves in the air, or the noise of traffic outside your car or home. Unless you pay attention to that transitory, fleeting memory, it essentially disappears from you forever.

2. Short-term memory:
   It is your memory of current events – the things that you are thinking about or looking at right now. In other words, it is the ability to actively hold the information in your mind in order to accomplish a task at hand. For example, a telephone number (without the need to have it repeated over and over), a list of grocery items, or a sequence of simple directions to complete a task.

   In fact, people use their short-term memories all the time without realizing it. Our short-term memory is supposed to have a limited finite capacity, typically between seven to ten things, which can be stored in the brain for 15 to 30 seconds.

3. Long-term memory:

It is established when you repeat or rehears those 7 to 10 items from the short-term memory, which are then transferred to the long-term memory. Long-term memory is likened to a limitless warehouse for storing our recollections for a long time. Long-term memory is considered the most and relevant kind of memories which allow us to go back to the past and predict the future. Just imagine to live a life without them is essentially no life at all!

Long-term memory relies on synaptic plasticity, that is, the formation of new synapses, or strengthening of existing and/or previous ones. Today, most neuro-scientists and researchers agree that synaptic plasticity is among the most important ways in which the brain stores information. Many studies have shown that the levels of neurotransmitters in the brain of individuals with Alzheimer's disease are reduced.

Memory is a very complex mental function. There are two major memory systems in the brain:

1. Explicit (or declarative) memory:

This allows us to consciously remember people, places and objects. This memory system also enables us to remember telephone numbers and addresses. If someone does not know the name of the capital of the U.S.A., you can tell them that it is Washington, D.C. Explicit memory works with the medical region of the temporal lobe of the brain.

2. Implicit (or non-declarative) memory:

This is the system which the brain uses for motor and perceptual skills that people do automatically such as driving a car, riding a bicycle, or swimming. As a contrast from explicit memory system, which interacts with and relies on higher, cognitive regions such as the medical region of the temporal lobes, implicit memory system depends on regions of the brain that respond to stimuli such as the amygdala, the cerebellum and the basal ganglia.

In other words, implicit memory system is usually well-preserved in old age, even in the early stages of Alzheimer's disease, and this is because the disease typically does not affect the amygdala, cerebellum and the basal ganglia. This explains why the persons with Alzheimer's who are unable to remember the names of loved ones or familiar places can still ride a bicycle, play the piano, read a book and swim.

It is unfortunate and heart-breaking that explicit memory for facts, events, people, etc., degrades early in the course of this illness. Thus, the patients are more likely to lose their more recent memories first, and the oldest ones are the last to go. This is the general pattern seen in people suffering from Alzheimer's in which their life is gradually erased in reverse order --- first the ability to recognize or recall the names of their most recent friends and the grandchildren. Then, the memory of their children disappears, and lastly, recollections of their spouses and siblings fade into the void.

When the electrical potentials pass repeatedly between two neurons, that particular synapse is strengthened. This is like walking in a wood; the more people walk along on the same path, the more the path becomes obvious and clear, and the more likely this particular path will be used again. If the neuronal pathways or circuits in the brain are not being used, they will degrade and degenerate, just like the walking path in the woods getting fainter and fainter when not being used.

Most of the memory activities are centered in the hippocampus, which is located in the temporal lobes on both sides of the brain. If one lobe is damaged, it is still possible for memory to function, but if both lobes are damaged, so is the capacity to remember. The hippocampus does not work alone; there are many connections between specific, relevant areas of the cortex and the hippocampus. When these connections are weakened and compromised, memories will fade and disappear; when they are strengthened and enhanced with stimulations, this helps to scribe the memories permanently into the architecture of the brain.

It is undeniable that one cannot learn when there is no memory. Learning and memory are the two most wonderful abilities of our mind. Learning is the process whereby we acquire new knowledge about the world and around us, and memory is the process whereby we retain the knowledge over time. Memory is the wonderful, remarkable and necessary "glue" that holds our psychic or mental life together. Without this amazing, unifying force, our consciousness will be degraded and broken into many, many fragments, and disconnected.

Age-related memory loss, also known as "benign senescent forgetfulness", can occur when you approach the middle age. Some researchers may consider it simply the early phase or precursor of Alzheimer's disease, but others, and I agree, regard it as a distinct entity in its own right.

Hippocampus can be very vulnerable; sometimes it can be damaged just by the lack of blood flow leading to cell death. Deficit in memory is the result from loss of synapses where neurons communicate. Many studies have demonstrated that the brain can re-grow synapses in the early stages of Alzheimer's disease if the affected person remains mentally active with appropriate brain stimulations. In the final stages of the disease, the neurons actually die. According to the recent neuro-scientific research, regular mental stimulation in older people can grow or form new dendrites to facilitate chemical signals to be sent from one neuron to another, strengthening and expanding the brain reserve.

The adult brains do make new neurons, called adult neurogenesis, which indeed does occur in the hippocampus throughout adult life. Hippocampal neurogenesis is enhanced by learning, estrogen and environmental enrichment. Conversely, stresses such as PTSD

(Post-traumatic Stress Disorder) can cause dendritic atrophy in the hippocampus according to research.

Experiments with rats have shown that housing the animals in a rich, stimulating environment increase their numbers of hippocampal synapses. It is generally accepted that a new memory requires a new neuron and the formation of a new synapse. Most recent studies by neuro-scientists, however, claim that this requirement of new neurons and new synapses is not absolute; it can be achieved by the strengthening of pre-existing synapses. In other words, synapses can be altered and reinforced by experience.

Very few dendrites, the receptive processes of neurons, are present at birth. During the first year of human life, there is an enormous increase in the number of dendrites, to the extent that each cortical neuron has enough dendrites to accommodate as many as 10,000 synapses with other neurons. This expansive, far-reaching pattern of synapses enables the human cortex to function as the center for learning, memory and reasoning.

In the Indonesian Island of Bali, there is a powerful myth of life cycles concerning memory, and it is just profound and mind-boggling. "Babies are born with no memory. They gather memories as they grow. As they get old, they have lost these memories so that they can be reborn again in a void".

Our identity is the sum of our memories. Alzheimer's disease is the worst thing that can happen to anyone who thinks because it takes them away.

THE LONG ORDEAL OF ALZHEIMER'S DISEASE

Somewhat unique to Alzheimer's disease, it is an unpredictable, ever-changing and kind of invisible chronic illness with mental and physical disabilities. Again, it is the worst thing that can happen to anyone who thinks. What is more powerless than the Alzheimer's sufferers? The feeling of powerlessness, helplessness and hopelessness must also be felt and experienced by the caregivers and family members. The pain and agony of this roller-coaster ride of hope and despair experienced by the patients and caregivers are indescribable.

In 1906, Dr. Alois Alzheimer in Frankfurt, Germany, was curious about one of his patients, named Auguste D. who lost her memories and did not know the names and use of certain familiar objects. His patient was also confused, exhibiting strange behaviors such as dragging her bed-sheets around during one of his home visits. Dr. Alzheimer performed an autopsy and his initial, obvious finding was an atrophic (small) brain due to cell death and other tissue damages.

Microscopically, he further found sticky deposits around the neurons which later researchers called amyloid plaques. Some tangles of Tau protein can also be found intracellularly in the brains of some Alzheimer's patients. Dr. Alois Alzheimer in 1907 gave the diagnosis of presenile dementia at the time, which was later named after him, the Alzheimer's disease.

Today, beta-amyloid plaques and Tau tangles are the two most important pathological, cellular features of Alzheimer's disease. There are different types of dementia, and Alzheimer's is the most common form making up about 65% to 70% of all dementia cases.

The symptoms of Alzheimer's are usually gradual and sometimes imperceptible, with memory noticeably impaired early in the illness. Typically, Alzheimer's disease is slowly and relentlessly progressive. Family and friends often do not notice the beginnings of language and motor problems; but as the dementing illness progresses, all of these symptoms will become apparent and noticeable. The impairment may have a stable period called "plateau" before reaching the late stages during which the impaired individual is incontinent and totally dependent on caregiver, unable to walk or talk or recognize anyone.

Vascular dementia:

This form of dementia is also called multi-infarct dementia, accounting for 30 to 35% of dementia cases. Depending on the areas of the brain being infarcted or damaged, it can affect memory, coordination or speech. Some vascular dementias may not get worse, become stabilized and even show improvement with successful rehabilitation if further strokes can be prevented. Some vascular dementias cannot be stopped and may co-exist with Alzheimer's disease.

Fronto-temporal dementia:

This form of dementia is not very common; it occurs when the frontal cortex is damaged from strokes or accidental head trauma. People with fronto-temporal dementia may show emotional apathy; they can exhibit behavioral disinhibition and socially inappropriate behaviors such as stealing, sexual assault, and inexplicable gambling habits.

Lewy body dementia:

It may be the third most common type of progressive dementia after Alzheimer's dementia and vascular dementia. This progressive brain disease is due to deposits of protein known as alpha-synuclein, collectively called Lewy bodies. Lewy bodies can form inside the synapses, causing the neurons to work less effectively and die.

This form of dementia is characterized by a progressive decline in mental abilities with apathy and loss of motivation. Patients may experience visual hallucinations and changes in alertness and attention. Parkinson's disease-like signs and symptoms may be observed with rigid muscles, slow movement and tremors. It may be difficult to distinguish between dementia of Alzheimer's disease and Lewy body dementia, but medical professionals can differentiate one from the other with diagnostic aids and the fluctuations of symptoms.

Dementia per se can be caused by different diseases and conditions besides Alzheimer's disease. Other neuro-degenerative disorders with a dementia component include Parkinson's disease, Huntington's disease, and multiple sclerosis. Some psychiatric disorders of depression and schizophrenia can have a component of dementia. Certain infections can cause dementia such as syphilis, meningitis and encephalitis.

Significant contributing factors of dementia include:

- Age – the older you get, the more likely you are to develop dementia
- Family history can be an important factor, especially the early-onset form of Alzheimer's disease
- Race/Ethnicity – older African Americas are twice more likely to have dementia than Caucasians
- Cardiovascular disease
- Traumatic Brain Injury – per advice of the Center for Disease Control and Prevention (CDC)

Special note: Certain infections can cause functional disruption of the brain, and the most recent example is the Corona pandemic. A recent landmark study of more than 200,000 survivors of post-COVID-19, commonly referred to as 'long haulers', has discovered that the participants in the study all suffered psychiatric or neurologic disability including brain-fog six months after the viral infection.

Vitamin B12 deficiency can lead to dementia, reversible with treatment. Thyroid disorders can cause dementia with some untreated cases. Virus such as AIDS can cause dementia sometimes when the HIV infects the brain. Poisoning with carbon monoxide and certain metals can cause dementia. Abuse of illicit drugs can cause temporary or permanent dementia in some cases. Brain tumors and brain traumas are known to cause dementia. Hypoxia and anoxia are fairly common causes of dementia, which is usually short-lived if corrective measures are quickly and appropriately instituted.

Alzheimer's disease is NOT a normal part of aging even though increasing age is the biggest known risk factor. Dementia is the clinical manifestation of years of accumulating neuropathology and progressive neuro-degeneration. The time of pre-clinical phase and the early stages is the window of golden opportunity for intervention, to optimize the brain for its functionality, to boost its neuronal networks, to stimulate the growth of new neurons and to help stave off age-related brain disorders.

In general, dementia is characterized by the following impairments:

- Impairment of memory, short-term and/or long-term
- Impairment of cognitive ability including language
- Impairment of social functioning and the ability to perform activities of daily living.

Sometimes the behavior of the individual with Alzheimer's disease can be very embarrassing, and the strangers often do not understand what is happening. Despite the growing awareness of Alzheimer's disease, many misconceptions remain. Nevertheless, there should be no stigma associated with having Alzheimer's disease or dementia.

Alzheimer's disease is a multi-dimensional chronic, age-related illness with many contributing and aggravating risk factors.

- The intercellular beta amyloid plaques and the intracellular neurofibrillary Tau tangles were found as evidence from post-mortem examinations of many Alzheimer's patients. Such tangles can occur in the absence of the amyloid plaques. Nevertheless, the presence of beta amyloid plaques and tau tangles serve to increase the risk for the development of Alzheimer's disease.

  However, some older people seem relatively resistant to the development of the disease, as researchers have discovered, despite an abundance of plaques and tangles in the brain confirmed by imaging, that their cerebral functions incredibly preserved even at advanced age. They are able to live without mental frailty and dysfunction. Thus, it is possible to resist and overcome the genetic and pathological forces, and indeed Alzheimer's disease is not an inevitable consequence of aging.

- ApoE4 gene variant:
  Genetic research at Duke University Medical Center in 1992 has shown that this variant of ApoE is associated with an increased risk for development of the sporadic form of Alzheimer's disease, also called late-onset Alzheimer's disease.

  People with a single copy of ApoE4 gene have a 3-fold greater risk of developing the disease; those with two copies, having inherited the gene from both parents, face a 12-fold greater risk, according to a group of researchers in a consortium led by the U.S. National Institute of Aging in 2016. In the absence of the genotype, ApoE, you are not immune to Alzheimer's disease.

The three variants of ApoE gene --- ApoE2, ApoE3 and ApoE4 --- code for different versions of a protein called apolipoprotein E, which aids the delivery of lipids and cholesterol to cells throughout the body. Therefore, the ApoE gene affects the risk of heart disease and stroke, but the involvement of the variant ApoE4 in Alzheimer's disease is still a mystery.

Some studies seem to suggest that the ApoE4 gene variant may enhance the deposition of beta-amyloid in the brain. This ApoE4 gene is probably more predictable for the early-onset form of Alzheimer's disease, accounting for less than 10% of all Alzheimer's cases; this early-onset form typically strikes the affected individuals well before the age 60.

- Oxidative stress:
  This is a "natural enemy" faced by all the cells in the body including neurons and glial cells of the brain. The biological damage is done by molecules called free radicals which are generated during biochemical reactions occurring in the body. In other words, oxidation is a process that occurs in the human body as the result of normal metabolism. Oxygen is absolutely necessary for life, but too much of it can be harmful. An oxidant is any compound that can accept electrons, or remove electrons from another compound. An antioxidant is a compound that donates electrons to prevent oxidation.

Normally, there is a mechanism in the body to maintain a balance or homeostasis with the removal of these free radicals. Free radicals are reactive oxygen species, ROS, which are molecules with unpaired electrons. Biochemically, molecules with unpaired electrons are unstable; they can steal or take electrons from the fatty acids that make up the cell membranes. When a molecule loses an electron, it is said to be oxidized. If the amount of free radicals produced and generated overwhelms the body's capacity to neutralize them, this will lead to oxidative stress, resulting in neuronal damage and eventual cell death.

The baseline levels of free radicals produced within the bodies from normal cellular metabolism can be managed physiologically because the normal human body is engineered to utilize naturally-occurring antioxidants to defend against oxidative damages. As one grows older, the cells' sensitivity to this kind of insult or injury goes up while the body's ability to heal afterward goes down or becomes less efficient.

Oxidative stress is significant and one of the widely accepted theories of aging and chronic diseases such as Alzheimer's disease. Its harmful effects on the body are pervasive; it causes the skin to lose its flexibility and accelerates the formation of wrinkles. Oxidative stress also increases inflammation in the arthritic joints, it raises the risk of cancers, it causes damages to the lens and retina of the eyes increasing the risk for cataract and retinopathy. Other adverse and harmful effects of oxidative stress includes the accumulation of atherosclerotic plaques on the inside of arterial walls making you more susceptible to stroke.

Brain tissues from Alzheimer's patients showed higher levels of oxidation than healthy, normal patients. Amyloid becomes sticky when oxidized, clumping together under oxidative stress. In 1995, researchers of structural molecular biology in Hamburg, Germany demonstrated that the Tau protein only coagulates when oxidized. The further found that when oxidation is prevented by antioxidants, tau protein will not coagulate. It seems clear that plaques and tangles tend to form under oxidative stress.

Unfortunately, we cannot abolish oxidative stress, but we can modulate it with mitigating factors to alleviate oxidative stress, postponing the onset of Alzheimer's or slowing its progression.

- Inflammation:
It is the body's natural response of the immune system to injury. There are different inflammatory markers in the body. One of them is CRP, C-reactive protein; it is a risk factor for heart disease and stroke. An increase in the levels of tumor necrosis factor alpha and Interleukin-6, two inflammatory agents in the Central Nervous System, seems to play a role in the age-related loss of memory and cognitive function.

Inflammation of the brain, according to researchers of neuroscience, promotes the formation of plaques and tangles, resulting in subsequent death of neurons. The harmful effects of inflammation on the brain are so vicious, insidious and destructive that the Canadian researchers have described Alzheimer's disease as "arthritis of the brain". Studies have shown that the levels of inflammatory mediators produced by the activated microglia of Alzheimer's brains are elevated and their concentrations are much lower in non-demented brains from normal aged individuals.

Some researchers have considered inflammation the root of almost all diseases, and a major culprit in accelerating the aging process and in causing age-related illnesses.

- Abdominal or visceral fats:
They are generally seen in people who are overweight and obese; they are also more and more visibly present in people who are not overweight and have normal body mass indexes. These visceral fats are very toxic, harmful and inflammatory. In 2008, data from a Permanente study of 7000 volunteers, aged 40 to 45, showed that those with bellies (abdominal fat) are more likely than those without abdominal fat to develop Alzheimer's disease later in life.

About 65 to 70% of the U.S. population are either overweight or obese. It is also becoming a public health problem in many developing countries. I call obesity "the evil master of health risks" because obesity causes multiple organ damages of the body with a wide variety of medical afflictions such as diabetes mellitus, cardiovascular diseases, sleep disorders and osteoarthritis, just to name a few.

One theory postulates that the visceral fats send damaging molecules through the blood stream to the brain. Many studies have shown that obesity is associated with increased levels of inflammatory markers and destructive inflammation of the body, compromising brain health and disrupting neuronal functions, thus, increasing the risk of developing Alzheimer's disease.

Head trauma (Traumatic Brain Injury):

- Any head injury hard enough to cause internal damage to the brain cells increases the risk for development of Alzheimer's disease and other forms of dementia, especially the insult to the head is repetitious. This is seen in certain sports such as boxing, American football, and soccer even with younger players in good health. In a study published in 2018 that included data on almost 2.8 million people in Denmark, collected over 36 years, researchers reported that traumatic brain injuries, TBIs were associated with a higher risk of dementia.

- Aluminum:
It is the third most abundant metal in the earth's crust. Epidemiological studies in England, France, Norway and Newfoundland had associated the high levels of aluminum in the drinking water to Alzheimer's disease. But the multi-national studies failed to show a clear conclusive causal connection between aluminum poisoning and dementia, according to some skeptical researchers.

At one time, the Island of Guam was found to have considerable aluminum deposits in the soil, resulting in high levels of aluminum concentration in the drinking water. During that time period, many people on the Island were showing symptoms similar to Alzheimer's and other dementia. When the aluminum contamination was removed from the sources of drinking water, the incidence of the illness dropped dramatically. Thus, it is reasonable to believe that there might be a correlation between Alzheimer's-type dementia and aluminum poisoning.

In 1965, there was a study done on rabbits, in which injections of aluminum salts were given into animals' brains. The researchers reported subsequent changes in the brain tissues resembling Alzheimer's in humans. Regardless of the lack of conclusive evidence of cause-and-effect, it is hard to deny or ignore the neurotoxic influences of aluminum poisoning.

- Amalgam dental fillings:

Amalgam is a mixture of mercury and silver and other metals. In 1990, some researchers claimed that the mercury in the dental fillings was released during chewing of food and then absorbed into the body. Over time, its accumulation in the study subjects could have caused Alzheimer's disease and other maladies in some of the participants due to its neurotoxic effects. Despite the reassurance by the American Dental Association that amalgam fillings had a safety record dating back more than a century, amalgam is nowadays replaced by non-amalgam materials.

- How about the mercury in some fish?

In the late 1950s and 1960s, more than 2000 people residing near Japan's Minamata Bay developed a crippling, debilitating disorder of the nervous system. After extensive investigation, ranging from analyses of the sludge and water in the Bay area, the fish in nearby water, the hair of local fishermen and their family, researchers conclusively proved that the illness was caused by mercury contamination from the local chemical plants.

It is incontrovertible that mercury is a neurotoxin, which can increase the risk for the development of Alzheimer's and other neuro-degenerative disorders. The U.S. FDA has issued guidelines in regards to the consumption of fish which have detectable levels of mercury, especially for pregnant women, women who are breast-feeding and women planning to conceive.

• Chronic sleep deprivation

Lack of adequate sleep or sleep deprivation is emerging, in our hectic society, as an important detrimental and contributing factor in the development of many illnesses including Alzheimer's disease because of its harmful effects on mental health and the immune system.

In fact, a 2017 meta-analysis of 27 studies found that chronic sleep deprivation raises the risk of cognitive impairment by 65%. Researchers from the National Health and Aging Trends Study at Brigham and Women's Hospital looked at data from 2,812 adults aged 65 and over, and concluded that chronic lack of adequate sleep, i e. getting five hours or less of sleep a night doubled the risk of dementia such as Alzheimer's compared to the recommended duration of seven to eight hours. The U.S. Sleep Foundation advises seven and eight hours a night for people 65 years old and over.

When young and healthy men were kept from sleeping even for one night, the levels of the biomarker tau for Alzheimer's disease were elevated according to a study published in Neurology. The human brain needs sufficient "down time" in order to eliminate metabolic and neurotoxic wastes. During sleep, new memories are consolidated and older memories are reinforced. The average American today sleeps less than six hours a night, about two hours less than a century ago. This is partly due to the proliferation of electric lights, followed by television, computers, smart phones and other sleep-robbers in our restless and hectic modern society.

According to Cedernaes, MD, PhD and colleagues of the Department of Neuroscience at Upsala University in Sweden, disrupted and insufficient sleep lead to increased levels of tau and beta-amyloid in the cerebral spinal fluids with an average of 17% increase. As we know, both tau and beta-amyloid are associated with an increased risk for Alzheimer's disease. It has become clearer that sleep may be an important lifestyle factor that can modulate the prospective risk of Alzheimer's disease. In short, too little sleep essentially sets the stage for some forms of dementia, especially among the middle-aged people.

Cigarette smoking:

• In addition to the polluted air you breathe and the hundreds of toxic chemicals in every cigarette, smoking is very harmful to your health because it is also a strong free-radical producer. Many of the noxious chemicals in the cigarette smoke react with oxygen to form millions of free radicals, causing extensive oxidative stress, especially in the lungs and the arterial walls.

Furthermore, it also activates the inflammatory cells, provoking more cellular damages. The oxidative stress and accompanying inflammation present a major risk factor for cardiovascular disease, cancer and neuro-degenerative disorders like Alzheimer's disease.

- Impaired hearing and vision

Unfortunately, we lose our auditory and visual acuity clarity as we become older, generally in a gradual manner. Being able to hear well increases alertness, and enhance brain stimulation and social interaction. Livingston and her colleagues were surprised to witness that hearing loss had a strong negative impact on cognitive health.

It is well established that hearing loss is associated with an increased risk of dementia, according to the Royal National Institute for Deaf People. Researchers from Northern Ireland studied 2,114 patients with a hearing impairment, each of whom was over 50, from the National Alzheimer's Co-ordinating Center. The team found that a third of participants who wore hearing aids had not developed dementia five years after their mild cognitive impairment, or MCI diagnosis. In contrast, this figure was only a fifth for those who did not use hearing aids.

Findings published in the Journal of Alzheimer's and Dementia supports the growing view that the use of hearing aids can help slow the onset of dementia and Alzheimer's. Through the use of hearing aids, the delay can be up to five years. Even though there is no cure for Alzheimer's and other neuro-degenerative forms of dementia, even a small beneficial effect of hearing loss treatment in delaying the disease can have significant implications for public health. Another study of 2,000 participants in the U.S. Health and Retirement Study revealed about 70% slower rate of cognitive decline after they started using hearing aids.

Researchers at the University of Manchester have found that vision, like hearing, is also crucial and important for brain health. They studied 2,000 older adults from the English Longitudinal Study of Aging after their successful cataract surgeries and found that improved or better vision slowed their cognitive decline by as much as 50%.

It is understandable and the experts agree that social isolation is often felt by the individuals with limited senses of hearing and vision; this in turn decreases intellectual and sensory stimulations for the brain. Correcting these two sensory problems and improving sensory perception allow the impaired, older individuals to participate in more brain activities, thus helping ward off or decelerate the development of Alzheimer's disease and other forms of dementia.

- Sedentary lifestyle:

Human beings are made to move, without movements and flow, our physical health and psychic life will suffer. Just imagine when an infant is born at delivery without any observable movements, it is a major concern for the mother, nursing staff and the attending physician.

We seem to be living in a fast-moving world, but ironically with unhealthy movements such as sitting behind the wheel in a moving or speeding car, cramped in the seat of a jet-plane traveling at 500 mph or faster, and staring at the constantly changing and moving scenes or electronic data on the screens of the computers, television and smart phones.

An inactive lifestyle with little or no exercise is extremely detrimental to the physical and mental health. Your musculoskeletal systems will weaken and stiffen resulting in atrophy and frailty. Your circulatory system will slow down with stasis. Your heart and lungs will have diminished functional capacities, delivering less nutrients and oxygen to different organs and tissues of the body, and the most critical one is the brain. Your mood will be depressed with suboptimal motivation, and your memories will be compromised.

The saying "use it, or lose it" is indeed very true. A sedentary lifestyle is no doubt a serious risk factor for the development of Alzheimer's disease and other health problems.

Social isolation and loneliness:

- Isolation and loneliness is entirely different from solitude, which is a voluntary and spiritual retreat as practiced by some religious groups including the Tibetan monks. I am not referring to individuals, young and older adults, who choose to live alone for a single lifestyle or for whatever their reason is. Perhaps, these individuals want to be able to do what they want without the influence and interference by other people.

According to the Government statistics, more and more older people in the U.S. are living alone, and the trend, unfortunately and woefully, will continue because the geriatric population is the fastest growing segment, not only in the U.S., but also in the world.

Feeling lonely or socially isolated can happen anywhere, even in a room full of people or at a party; the plight of social isolation is unhealthy, physically, mentally and spiritually. It is a set-up for senility and for everything that can go wrong with the body and mind. Human beings are highly social species; we are meant to live in tribes, families and communities.

Social isolation is a disconnection. When you are disconnected or feeling disconnected, you find no meaning or purpose in your life. You lose connections to your spouse, your family, your friends, your work, or really anything beyond yourself. Without an enriched surroundings coupled with the lack of social interactions and the absence of different sensory stimulations for the brain, there is no question that social isolation and loneliness serve as a strong risk factor for the development of Alzheimer's.

It is my personal opinion that chronic illnesses such as Alzheimer's disease, to some degree, can be directly and also indirectly related to the breakdown of the family units and the weakening and ultimately dissolving of the family bonds that once extended from birth to death among several generations under the same roof.

Alzheimer's disease has grown considerably in proportion to these changing patterns of our modern-day society. The anti-dote to the withdrawal from life "in this disconnection syndrome of Alzheimer's sufferers will not be found, wholly and solely, in the technologies of medical science despite three or more decades of intense search for a cure of the disease. We, humanity, must do some serious soul-searching with increased social awareness and positive cultural changes in our battle against this horrible, dementing illness.

• Depression:

This negative emotion and mental disorder along with its clinical manifestation has reached an epidemic proportion in our stressful society. Many studies have revealed that depression predates the onset of Alzheimer's disease, and constitutes a distinct risk factor.

There are many observational studies showing the prevalence of depression among Alzheimer's patients, ranging from 20 to 40%. However, the link between depression and Alzheimer's disease is not clear: Is depression an emotional response to the terrible losses caused by the illness? Or, the depression itself makes the individuals more susceptible to the development of Alzheimer's? This takes us back to the proverbial question: "Which is first, chicken or egg"?

It is understandable that depression can happen to the caregiver also in this long, grueling journey with his or her impaired loved one. Both the caregiver and the patient should not hesitate to seek professional intervention for mental health.

Both the caregiver and the patient should be aware of some straight-forward simple causes of depression such as nutritional deficiency in a

Wholistic approach. Deficit or deficiency of B12, B6, folate, vitamin D, omega-3 fatty acids and niacin can lead to depression and mental dysfunction, according to many studies showing their associations.

- Post-chemotherapy brain fog:

Colloquially known as "chemo brain" by the patients; every year, there are anywhere between 650,000 and 700,000 cancer patients receiving chemotherapy in the U.S. During and after the treatment, up to 75% of patients experience confusion, lapses in memory and attention, and difficulty concentrating, in addition to the many side effects of the chemotherapy such as nausea and vomiting, diarrhea, fatigue, hair loss, anemia, insomnia, infection, tinnitus, alteration of taste and smell, leukopenia, thrombocytopenia, easy bruising and bone-marrow suppression. With the brain fog, patients can have trouble multitasking, or feeling mentally "slower" than usual.

Fortunately, most of the patients fully recover from the phenomena of cognitive and memory impairments within a year, but about 30% of them continue to experience the "brain fog" for months to years after their chemotherapy is completed, increasing their risk for the development of Alzheimer's disease.

Researchers, including cognitive psychologists, neuroscientists and oncologists, supported in large part by the National Cancer Institute, have been focusing on the genetics of susceptibility to cancer-based cognitive impairment and on the impact of different chemotherapies on cognition and memory. Many tend to dismiss the possibility that chemotherapy could be causing cognitive and memory issues because chemotherapies were not believed to cross the blood-brain barrier. The impairments can undermine patient's quality of life, yet for many it is so subtle that it is not easily detectable by the oncologists.

However, several animal studies in the past decade showed that chemotherapy drugs could pass through the blood-brain barrier. And neuro-imaging studies of patients after chemotherapies demonstrated that their neural networks had been altered, making the brains work much harder to do the same tasks.

But how exactly chemotherapy treatments affect the brain is still under investigation.

Different mechanisms for possible explanation include damages to the DNA, compromised DNA repair, oxidative stress, inflammation, dysfunction of the white matter, reduced blood flow and poor signaling and receptivity.

Studies by D. Shelli Kesler of the Livestrong Cancer Institute at the University of Texas in Austin showed that chemotherapy ages you faster, including your brain, accelerating neuro-degeneration. The brains of cancer patients who had chemotherapy looked older than their chronological age. Dr. Kesler further observed that the brains of these chemotherapy patients, upon imaging, have similar connectivity patterns to the brains of people suffering from Alzheimer's disease (Alzheimer's and Dementia, Vol 9, No. 1, 2017). In addition, neuroimaging studies of brain volume suggest chemotherapy leads to a decrease in both gray matter and white matter.

Since not all cancer patients undergoing chemotherapy experience cognitive decline with impaired memory, it is imperative to find out who is most at risk, to have a health-service psychologist on the treatment team with the baseline of patient's mental status on file, taking the preventive approach.

With its multiple adverse reactions and side effects, and potential toxicities on the CNS including the brain, some patients will not consider chemotherapy as part of their cancer treatment program, and their fear and concern are quite understandable. Consideration to go through chemotherapy must be taken seriously with a multi-pronged, wholistic approach with the dignity and quality of patients life as an integral part of the equation.

• Hypertension:

This is a common medical condition, and a serious risk factor for many diseases including Alzheimer's. It is a "silent killer" affecting the body

With many consequences including the damages to the brain. Hypertension is the leading cause of strokes, both mini and major. Up to 50% of the Alzheimer's sufferers showed multiple mini-strokes, called ischemic infarcts. These lesions with decreased oxygen and nutrients to the brain serve to heighten the risk for the development of Alzheimer's disease.

A recent study has found that young adults with history of high blood pressure often show signs of brain shrinkage with decreased gray matter in certain areas of the brain. The 423 study participants were between the ages 19 to 40 and underwent MRI scans. The findings were significant and countered the assumption that brain shrinkage (atrophy) happens only in older people with hypertension. "There is a gradual change that probably occurs throughout life and ends when people have a stroke or cognitive decline", researcher H. Lina Schaare from the Max Planck Institute in Leipzig, Germany, tells the New York Times. "A blood pressure around 130 in young people is not necessarily benign".

- Atherosclerosis:

The condition presents a serious and dangerous threat both to the heart and the brain. It is the underlying pathogenesis in a group of disorders collectively termed Cardiovascular Disease (CVD) which includes coronary disease, myocardial infarction, pulmonary and cerebral infarction. CVD is the number one cause of death in the U.S. Cerebral infarction is a stroke, sometimes called a 'brain attack', which is the result of two events inside the head: a sudden decrease of blood supply to a part of the brain, or bleeding in the brain. This is a medical emergency due to a sudden change in the brain functions. According to the American Heart Association, someone in the U.S. suffers a stroke every 40 seconds, and one life is lost every 4 to 5 minutes due to a major stroke.

The clogged blood vessels cannot transport adequate blood supply, thus reducing the levels of needed oxygen and nutrients to the organs and tissues of the body. A blockage or rupture of a blood vessel at a strategic location of the brain can give the sudden appearance of dementia, increasing the risk of Alzheimer's in slow progression. Nothing needs oxygen more than the brain, which accounts for only 2% of the body weight but demands 20% of the available oxygen.

- Diabetes Mellitus:

  This insidious but prevalent and terrible disease affects millions of people worldwide, and more and more new cases are being diagnosed everyday.

  It is a microvascular disease with multiple systemic organ damages; lesions in the microvasculature reduce oxygen and nutrient supply to the eyes, kidneys and the brain.

  Hyperinsulinemia, a chronic condition of elevated level of insulin in the blood, can have profound, far-reaching and serious detrimental effects on the brain, making hyperinsulinemia a significant risk factor for the development of Alzheimer's disease. Cognitive impairment due to repeated hypoglycemic episodes are stressful and harmful to the brain.

  A researcher/pathologist at Brown University, Suzanne Delamonte called Alzheimer's disease type-3 diabetes because it affects the brain and has many molecular and biochemical features common with type-2 diabetes, which is a major risk factor for Alzheimer's disease. In fact, the connections between glucose handling, insulin signaling and Alzheimer's are so strong that many researchers refer to Alzheimer's as "diabetes of the brain".

ANTI-ALZHEIMER'S STRATEGIES

Alzheimer's disease is a multi-dimensional, multi-causal condition, which is influenced by many, different factors, and most of those we can have some control to modify the course of this long illness. Hundreds and thousands of prescriptions have been written for millions of Americans and patients worldwide without certain efficacy, mostly as an attempt to placate patients' family members and friends and the frustrated caregivers who feel compelled to "do something".

There is no cure for Alzheimer's at this time. Researchers are still scrambling to find a way to show or stop the progression of this disease, let alone offer a cure, despite several decades of research and trials. The desire and interest to explore and try alternative approaches and therapeutic intervention are growing, as frustration about the medical model is spreading. In fact, some in the pharmaceutical industries have already given up the search of a therapeutic agent for a cure.

Nothing is enough to describe the tragically slow and agonizing events affecting individuals with this dementing illness. They seem to lose themselves gradually over time, forgetting their family members and friends, and in the end, becoming totally dependent and bed-ridden, and wholly disconnected from the world around them.

Please be reminded that dementia is not a normal part of getting older. Aging with Alzheimer's disease may be inevitable for up to 50% of the people 85 and older, but there are promising strategies and neuroprotective measures you can use and follow to avoid its perdition to retain your lucid mind, dignity and quality of life with some independence.

The so-called late-onset or sporadic Alzheimer's disease is usually slow-progressing, and unpredictable. There is a long gap or large window of opportunity for us to study and address what happens inside the brain, and potentially to slow down, halt, or even reverse it during the early stages of the illness.

We are going to look at the different factors that can help minimize and decrease the risk for the development of the disease and may change its course.

Knowing that you have the gene variant for Alzheimer's, it simply gives you a certain probability of something happening down the line, but it tells you very little about your near future. Many studies have shown that modification and suppression of gene expression is possible with environmental and other factors. The followings are the anti-Alzheimer's strategies, a multi-modal intervention within your power:

1. You can start with your kitchen where you prepare and cook your foods. Many studies have shown possible neurotoxicity of aluminum, even though the cause-and-effect linkage has not been conclusively established. Just because some researchers are expressing doubts and are not convinced by the evidences against aluminum, why should you take any chance on your brain. After all, it is your life.

   As a preventive strategy, avoid drinking beverages out of aluminum cans,
   Stop using antacids that contain aluminum, stop certain brand of baking
   Powder that has aluminum, and replace all your aluminum utensils in the
   Kitchen with those made of glass, ceramic or stainless steel.

Furthermore, some brand of table salts may contain
    aluminum silicate as an additive
With most of the mineral and trace elements stripped.
    Personally, I
Like the sea salt, which has many minerals and elements the
    body needs in
Trace amounts.

Some studies have shown possible link between aluminum poisoning in the drinking water and Alzheimer's type of CNS disorder. One study was done on the Island of Guam, and the others were done in England, France, Norway and Newfoundland. Despite the lack of unequivocal correlation between aluminum poisoning and dementia, avoiding and alleviating the accumulation of aluminum in the body is a wise strategy to protect yourself against any possible neurotoxic effect of aluminum on your brain.

2. Get rid of any amalgam dental fillings because some of the older folks might still have them from their dentists years ago. Nowadays, there are non-amalgam dental materials for replacement to avoid the neurotoxic effects of mercury on your body, the brain in particular.

3. Be a seafood (fish) lover and educated consumer about the levels of mercury in certain fish. The U.S. FDA has issued guidelines in this regard. There are basically a few fish you should be concerned about due to their high levels of mercury; they include king mackerel, marlin, orange roughy, swordfish, tilefish and bigeye tuna.

Most of the healthy, fatty fish are common, and they include salmon, sardine, mackerel, catfish, pollock, tilapia and many others. Seafood with fish is a wonderful choice for a low-carbohydrate diet; carbohydrate provides only four calories of energy per gram, where as fats provide nine calories of energy per gram. The omega-3 fatty acids of fish provide the body with tremendous health benefits, especially for your brain. Fatty fish such as salmon, sardines, trout, tuna, herring, anchovy and mackerels are readily available and are excellent sources of the heart-healthy and brain-healthy omega-3 fatty acids.

Healthy fats are very important for good health, and they facilitate the absorption of fat-soluble vitamins, namely, A, D, E and K. They serve as essential building blocks for the structure of cell membranes and plasma membranes. They are also structural components of myelin, the protective sheath that surrounds the neurons and facilitates effective neuronal communications

The brain is about 60% fat and most of that is docosahexaenoic acid, DHA, which is a polyunsaturated omega-3 fatty acid. DHA is very vital and crucial for optimal functioning of the brain besides its critical role in the development of the fetal brain and spinal cord. In fact, DHA is such a key structural component in the brain that it accounts for as much as 40% of the fatty acids in the cell membrane of neurons. These specialized fats, called fatty acids, are extremely important and helpful for the brain and body. Here is just a few things they do:

- They serve as rich sources of energy
- They facilitate the absorption of fat-soluble vitamins and important nutrients including vitamins A, D, E, K, and carotenoids such as lutein, lycopene and beta-carotene.
- They serve as essential building blocks for cell membranes and plasma membranes.
- They provide insulation and protective linings for vital organs, e.g. lung surfactant.
- They serve as structural component of myelin of the neurons, facilitating effective neuronal communications and signaling.

- They are required for the production of bile which aids in proper digestion.

Studies have demonstrated that low levels of DHA in the hippocampus may have a role in the cognitive decline in the elderly and Alzheimer's patients. Other recent neuro-scientific research has shown that a low-carbohydrate diet with increased intake of DHA from seafood seem to delay the development of Alzheimer's disease. In fact, Alzheimer's patients exhibit lower levels of DHA in their plasma and brain. Epidemiologically, researchers have found that increase DHA via dietary intake of seafood can reduce the risk of Alzheimer's disease with less cell death and apoptosis, and enhanced signaling pathways. This is probably due to the ability of DHA to increase the production of anti-inflammatory molecules and to reduce the viscosity of the blood, thus improving blood flow and preventing strokes.

Currently, the biggest nutritional deficiency in the Western countries is the low intake of omega-3 polyunsaturated fatty acids in the form of fresh fish, not the fried variety. If you have an allergy to seafood, you can obtain and increase your omega-3 fatty acids from plant sources, such as flax seeds, chia seeds and walnuts.

According to several studies from Harvard Medical School, babies delivered by women with higher blood levels of DHA were more attentive to stimuli. For the next six months, the same babies scored higher on tests of cognition than babies born to women with lower levels of DHA. In 2009, scientists at Sweden's Gothenburg University reported that 15-years-old boys and girls who ate fish at least twice a week scored higher on intelligence tests than their non-fish-eating peers. From the standpoint of dietary factor, fish is the single most important for cognitive health, especially in Alzheimer's disease. Thus, to avoid and minimize the development of Alzheimer's, fish is the most important dietary factor, according to recent Harvard studies.

Some words of caution: There is a risk associated with eating raw fish or shellfish, especially if you are immune-compromised or suffering from inflammatory bowel diseases. Sometimes consumers become ill with foodborne illnesses by Salmonella and Vibrio vulnificus.

According to the researchers at BarcelonaBeta Brain Research Center (BBRC) in Bacelona, Spain, they studied the middle-aged adults who were at higher genetic risk for the development of Alzheimer's disease, that is, they had two ApoE4 alleles but received a high intake of DHA exhibited more resistance to pathologic structural changes in their brains. Their brain scans showed much less atrophy and cortical thinning on neuro-imaging

4. Protecting your head at all times to avoid any trauma or injury to the head, minor or major. For the sports-minded and younger population, the concerns are the contact sports, such as American football and boxing. Others, to a lesser extent, include soccer and wrestling. For the older adults, it is important to wear seat belts at all times when riding as a passenger or driving behind the wheel. Seat belts, coupled with air-bags, do save lives and minimize direct head trauma in case of an accident or sudden, forceful stopping.

Traumatic Brain Injury (TBI) is defined as any injury or trauma to the brain due to an external force. It is estimated that more than 1.7 million Americans a year suffer Traumatic Brain Injury resulting in changes in the brain structure and function, as well as thinking and memory struggles (or difficulties) which can be either temporary or permanent. The symptoms of TBI are variable, depending on the extent and frequency of the injury; they include, but not limited to, loss of consciousness, nausea or vomiting, headache and fatigue, loss of balance, blurred vision and impaired speech.

According to the most recent neuroscientific studies, TBI and Alzheimer's disease appear to affect the brain in similar ways. Researchers found similar cortical thinning in patients with TBI and Alzheimer's disease. Cortical thinning is often associated with declines in attention, memory and speech, as well as impaired abilities to make decisions, integrate new information and adapt behavior to new situations. Their MRI scans showed similar deterioration in the gray and white matters of the brain in the studies. All of these findings do not definitively establish a cause-and-effect relationship between TBI and Alzheimer's, but both conditions share similar trajectory.

If you enjoy and are able to do bike-riding, wear your helmets as a precautionary measure against possible direct head impact. It is my advice that for individuals with Alzheimer's even in the early stages, it is best to refrain from bicycling due to the unpredictable nature of the disease; instead, go for a walk or a swim, but never alone.

5. Adequate intake of quality protein is important for good health, especially among the elderly. It is true and commonly known that muscles are made predominantly of protein, but it is also an integral part of hair, skin, nails, blood vessels, tendons, ligaments and even bones. The antibodies of the immune system is also made from protein, as are many hormones such as insulin and growth hormone. The enzymes that regulate and control many biochemical reactions inside the body are protein.

The recommended range for protein intake as a percentage of the total calories for an average adult is 15 to 30%, according to the U.S. Institute of Medicine; and the recommended

Daily Allowance for protein is 0.36 gram per pound of body weight.

Protein is especially important for older people facing the decrease of muscle mass with aging. Sufficient protein intake along with appropriate exercise help to maintain muscle tissue and insulin sensitivity, and reduce the risk of physical frailty in the elderly. Beef, pork, lamb and poultry are excellent sources of good-quality protein. One can also obtain plant-based protein from beans.

Unfortunately, many people in the seniors choose to eat the fried versions of meat, chicken in particular due to the convenience, reasonable costs, and the addictive flavor in the starchy wraps coated and deep-fried in flour-based batter. Deep-frying of any type of food is not a healthy way of cooking, and it is prudent and wise to resist fried foods for the sake of your body and mind.

6. Making sure that there is adequate level of vitamin B12 (cyanocobalamin) in your body. Vitamin B12 is necessary for proper functioning and formation of myelin in the Central Nervous System (the brain and the spinal cord). In fact, many studies have shown that low B12 level is an important risk factor for loss of brain volume among older people, and the serum B12 status may be an early marker of brain atrophy, according to the research.

Sometimes, severe vitamin B12 deficiency, also known as pernicious anemia, is misdiagnosed as dementia because signs and symptoms of B12 deficiency include depression, memory loss, decreased cognitive function and peripheral neuropathy.

Gastric acids are required for the absorption of vitamin B12 from foods. This actually is a problem, often unnoticed, for many older people, who have been taking either OTC antacids and/or prescriptions for proton pump inhibitors such as Nexium and Prilosec for conditions like reflux esophagitis, dyspepsia and peptic ulcer disease.

This low gastric acid environment, iatrogenic, and the subsequent decrease in vitamin B12 absorption can be exacerbated by the tendency of the senior population to consume fewer foods that are rich in vitamin B12 such as red meat (grass-fed), and shellfish (oysters, clams mussels and scallops). Many of them living on their own with limited budgets are more likely to choose convenient and cheaper carbohydrates such as noodles, pasta and spaghetti which are easier to prepare and chew, rather than cooking a meal of healthy fat and protein for themselves.

The geriatric group of our society has a special need for vitamin B12; it is highly soluble in water and there should not be any concern about toxicity

Below 2,000 mcg a day, even though it is above the Government's Recommended Daily Allowance. The best and fastest way to raise low blood levels of vitamin B12 is by subcutaneous or intra-muscular injections when necessary.

7. Getting sufficient folic acid (or folate) is important for good health, especially the brain. It is one of the B-vitamins and you can find it in abundance in dark, green leafy vegetables such as broccoli, spinach and kale. Many fruits, beans and nuts are also good sources of folate.

In 1965, Landmark studies published in the Lancet, the prestigious British medical journal documented that 66% of the mother in the studies who gave birth to babies with brain and spinal cord malformations were deficient in folic acid. A follow-up report two years after the stunning Lancet publication of the studies in 1965 suggested that folic acid deficiencies might also be linked to dementia and brain atrophy --- the shrinkage typically seen in Alzheimer's disease.

Furthermore, in the study by researchers at Oxford University Project to Investigate Memory and Aging (the OPTIMA study), they reported that low blood levels of folic acid seem to be a significant risk factor for the development of Alzheimer's disease and brain atrophy. The neuroprotective effects of folic acid on human development are clear and convincing; this nutrient, which has such a dramatic impact at the beginning of life, may guard the end of life as well.

If your diet consists of 75 to 80% of fruits and vegetables, your body should have adequate levels of folic acid. If this is not the case with your lifestyle, folic acid should be included in your judicious supplementation of multiple vitamins. With its neuroprotective benefits, you have nothing to lose but everything to gain.

8. Don't be afraid of cholesterol, which has had a bad and scary reputation for quite some time. And the tide is turning because more and more researchers and neuro-scientists are finding out that cholesterol is critical and necessary for brain health and cognitive function. In fact, cholesterol should be the brain's good friend, if not the best, because the lack of

Cholesterol supply to the neurons can impair neuro-transmission and synaptic plasticity, leading to neuro-degeneration.

Like fatty acids, cholesterol is one of the building blocks of myelin in the brain. In a typical adult body, the brain accounts for 2% of the total body weight, but it holds 25% of the body's cholesterol. The human body does manufacture cholesterol for itself, but sometimes it may not produce enough to meet the body's needs because cholesterol is such an integral part of many body's structures such as cells and tissues. Cholesterol is also an integral component of many biochemical processes in the body.

Myelin is made mostly out of cholesterol, and adequate amount of cholesterol is necessary to create and maintain the myelin sheath of the nerves. Otherwise, the neurons will "short out" just like the ungrounded electrical wires; the outcome of neurons misfiring and failing to communicate effectively with other neurons will be memory loss, confusion and behavioral changes as seen in people with Alzheimer's disease.

Cholesterol is the raw material for endogenous production of vitamin D through interaction of sunlight with the skin. Cholesterol is also required for the synthesis of steroid hormones which include testosterone and estrogen. The health benefits of testosterone and estrogen are discussed later on in this chapter. Another wonderful benefit is the production of co-enzyme Q-10, which is created during the synthesis of cholesterol. Co-enzyme Q10 is a well-known popular antioxidant with many health benefits such as for the heart and brain. Last but not least, cholesterol is an essential component of bile salts which aid the digestion of foods and absorption of fat-soluble vitamins and phytonutrients.

If you are still skeptical and concerned about cholesterol, as a defense, there is no direct evidence that cholesterol by itself blocks the coronary or cerebral arteries, causing myocardial infarction (heart attack) or cerebrovascular accident (stroke). Just because cholesterol is found in the plaques inside the arteries in atherosclerosis does not mean cholesterol is the culprit because there are other things that can cause damages to the endothelial lining of the artery, and there are other factors that can contribute to the event of a heart attack. Through recent research, we have discovered that it is actually saturated fat, not dietary cholesterol, that increases our blood cholesterol.

Many studies have demonstrated that people with normal blood level of cholesterol die from heart attack just as often as people with elevated level of cholesterol. In essence, blood cholesterol level cannot predict a heart attack! Similarly, cholesterol cannot predict a stroke either, because there are many other risk factors such as diabetes, hypertension, lack of exercise, etc. Interestingly, researchers have found that the levels of cholesterol in the cerebrospinal fluid (CSF) of people with Alzheimer's disease are lower than that of normal, healthy people.

9. Eating a hard-boiled egg 3 to 5 times a week. Eggs were once considered "brain food"; for some vague and unfounded reason, they went out of favor for a while. Many people and consumers are confused by eggs because of the confusing information out there over a decade ago when the health professionals and nutritionists were recommending people to stay away from eggs. This is mainly because there was such a misunderstanding between dietary cholesterol and cardiovascular disease, and foods with high cholesterol such as eggs would increase blood cholesterol levels and then augment your chance of cardiovascular disease, which is the leading cause of death in the U.S.

Eggs are a brain food indeed. In 2015, Dietary Guidelines for Americans advised that there was no proof that dietary cholesterol was a direct contributor to an increase in blood cholesterol levels. In fact, we must pay attention to saturated fats, trans fats, and added sugars instead. So, eat the entire egg, egg white and yolk, and do not eat it with bacon and sausages.

If you avoid the yolk, you are missing some of the important nutrients; besides being a good source of protein, which can help cell growth, build lean muscles, and help keep you feeling full longer, eggs also contain a large dose of vitamin D, vitamin B12, vitamin A, vitamin E, zinc, and choline.

Eggs are a good source of cholesterol and choline, which is required for the production of neurotransmitter, acetylcholine in the brain. Researchers have found several neurotransmitters, particularly acetylcholine, are deficient in people suffering from Alzheimer's disease, and increasing the levels of acetylcholine will relieve the symptoms of Alzheimer's.

Eggs also are a good source of important trace elements such as copper, selenium, manganese and phosphorus. In a large observational study published in the British Medical Journal Heart', researchers investigated and surveyed the study participants about their frequency of egg consumption, and found that people who ate up to seven eggs a week --- one egg a day --- were significantly less likely to develop cardiovascular disease than participants who did not eat eggs.

One can find various amounts of free choline and choline esters in most foods, but most abundant in foods of animal origins such as eggs and livers. Free choline and choline esters are very abundant in human breast milk; all infant formulas nowadays have content of choline compounds to levels similar to human breast milk.

Many studies have demonstrated that choline deficiency can lead to cognitive and memory deficits, and adequate levels of choline can help improve memory and learning by increasing the rate of synthesis of neurotransmitters. Choline is also involved in the creation of cell membrane components, called phospholipids; phospholipids can help repair and protect neurons whose membranes have been damaged.

Undoubtedly, the three nutrients of cholesterol, choline and vitamin B12 are extremely critical and indispensable for structure and function of a healthy brain, especially for older adults with Alzheimer's disease. I call them collectively "neuroprotective triad".

10. Do yourself a big favor and quit smoking cigarette. And if you do not smoke, try to avoid second- hand smoking. Most people are familiar with the heightened risk of lung cancer associated with cigarette smoking, but unaware of, or ignoring, or not knowledgeable about the many other serious health consequences of smoking.

Besides the much greater chance of developing lung cancers than non-smokers, smokers, regular or heavy, have at least three times greater than non-smokers the chance of dying of a heart attack. Emphysema and other respiratory infections are more common among smokers. The chance of premature death from any cause is also much higher with smokers, as compared with non-smokers.

Cigarette smoking tends to accelerate the aging processes of the body; smokers are more likely to develop facial wrinkles and a haggard look. Apart from smokers themselves, many studies have shown that children of smoking parent(s) suffer higher incidences of chronic obstructive pulmonary disease, such as bronchitis and emphysema.

Cigarette contains hundreds of harmful chemicals, and the most notorious one is nicotine, which is highly addictive and a powerful vaso-constrictor. Its property of vasoconstriction can increase blood pressure and decrease blood flow, raising the risk of stroke directly and the risk of the development of Alzheimer's disease indirectly.

The air-pollutants in the smoke and the toxic chemicals in the cigarettes greatly increase the oxidative activities throughout the body, with the elevated levels of free radicals overwhelming and tilting the body's equilibrium. In other words, cigarette smoking is certainly the most insidious culprit for free-radical damages to the body, the brain in particular. The hundreds of free radicals in a single puff of cigarette smoke also trigger inflammatory cells, adding more toxins and stress to the body. In fact, one can measure the damaged, oxidized fragments of DNA from Cigarette smoking excreted in the urine as 8-hydroxy-deoxyguanosine (8-OHdG).

11. Stay well-hydrated. Most of us tend to take water for granted because it is so freely and readily available everywhere. Ironically, many of us are not drinking enough water, and chronic dehydration is actually quite common. We are not aware of, or do not realize the paramount importance of adequate water intake for our physical and mental health.

Nowadays, with the constant advertisements and ubiquitous sensual bombardments about manufactured beverages such as beer, coffee, sodas and juices, most people are paying less and less attention to simple, pure water. In fact, most, if not all of those commercial beverages advertised contain dehydrating ingredients which deplete the water content of the body, though unintentionally.

The human body is about 70% water, whereas the human brain is at least 75% water and is very sensitive to any degree of dehydration at cellular levels. Water is not just a simple, inert substance; it is life-giving and life-sustaining. Each cell of the human body is about 75% water, which is critical in the production of electrical energy for all brain functions, including thinking. One of the first signs of dehydration is 'brain fog' --- being unable to concentrate and having difficulty remembering things.

A study by mental health researchers of 3,327 participants have found that those who drank two glasses or less of plain water per day reported higher levels of depression than those who drank five glasses or more each day. Water and mood are so connected that even very mild dehydration --- losing just one percent of total body water can cause depression, according to a study published in The Journal of Nutrition.

As we get older, we lose the sharpness, acuity and precision of our senses including hearing, vision, taste, smell and thirst. Due to the gradual loss of thirst, more and more people fail to drink water adequately; this phenomenon has profound, detrimental effects on the elderly, in particular, both physically and mentally. To make the situation worse, people often confuse the sensation of thirst with the feeling of hunger. So, instead of drinking water, which is essentially an appetite suppressant, they eat foods adding more calories to their weight and becoming more dehydrated.

Coincidentally, many patients with Alzheimer's disease have impaired olfactory sense. In fact, worsening of olfaction is often used as a marker for disease progression. Keep in mind that zinc deficiency is known to cause reduced senses of taste and smell.

Studies by Phillips and Associates have shown that after 24 hours of water deprivation, the elderly participants still do not realize or recognize that they are thirsty. Other studies published in the Lancet have supported the conclusion that the thirst mechanism is gradually lost in the elderly with aging.

The human body has not stored water to draw from in the case of dehydration; that is why we must drink water regularly and throughout the day. If the body weight is 120 pounds, take half of that in ounces of water, i.e. you need an average of 60 oz of water over a 24-hour period for that body weight so that the body can function optimally. This is equivalent to seven to eight 8-oz glasses of water a day. Certain conditions such as increase perspiration, fever, hot surroundings like high temperatures, and strenuous or even normal physical activities, will increase your need for water beyond the normal average amount.

If an older individual has heart problems or kidney diseases, one must increase the water intake slowly if dehydrated, and with the supervision of your physician. It is prudent and necessary to consult the attending doctor if fluid restriction has been ordered, and to maintain records of the daily input or intake of fluid and the output. Otherwise, caregiver should not wait for the patient with Alzheimer's disease to let you know he or she is thirsty.

An important scientific paper by Ephraim Katchalski-Katzir of the Weitzmann Institute demonstrated that proteins and enzymes function more efficiently in solutions of lower viscosity, i.e. they need adequate water in their immediate milieu to work optimally. The most significant complication and consequence of dehydration is the loss of the necessary essential amino acids in the production of neuro-transmitters.

Therefore, chronic dehydration can disrupt neuronal function and cause neurological damage to the brain because the raw materials become less available for the brain to make neuro-transmitters.

Our body and brain are run and maintained on a fine-tuned system, and dehydration throws the balance off. When necessary nutrients like salt becomes too concentrated in the blood, one can experience "altered mental states" and if dehydration continues without treatment, it can cause seizures. Furthermore, chronic dehydration is associated with shrinking brain tissue and reduced brain volume, according to findings of studies published in JAMA Psychiatry.

Chronic dehydration can also lead to a metabolic problem of acidity. Water in sufficient supply washes away acidic buildup out of the cells and makes the interior alkaline --- a healthier physiological state for optimal bodily functions --- a pH of 7.4. The DNA in the nucleus of a cell is sensitive to the corrosive effects of an acidic environment, rendering it more susceptible to damages or changes. It is easy to understand that adequate water intake with normal hydration status has definite neuroprotective effects for the brain.

The mind-body connection is significant and undeniable, and a dehydrated body will worsen short-term memory, cause poor job performance, impair alertness and working memory. There are many mental symptoms of dehydration, some can be obvious, and some subtle:

- Confusion
- Increased irritability, or having a short fuse
- Mental slowness
- Fatigue
- Headache
- Difficulty and/or inability to concentrate
- Ruminating
- Unexplained sadness
- Anxiety

12. Keeping your blood pressure readings within normal limits. Hypertension is a common public health challenge, nicknamed "a silent killer", which exerts profound, insidious, detrimental effects on the entire body, notably the heart, the kidneys and the brain.

Approximately 30% of the U.S. adults have the diagnosis of hypertension; furthermore, at least another 30% of American adults have pre-hypertension. Even though the cause of hypertension is mostly unknown, idiopathic or essential, many cases are due to identifiable and underlying correctable conditions.

In contrast to the relatively high prevalence in the U.S., many non-westernized and developing countries and remote populations have a low prevalence of hypertension and do not experience an increase in blood pressure with age. According to many epidemiological studies, their protection from hypertension is often attributed to a low salt intake, a high potassium intake, being physically active and generally higher plant and fish consumption. Migration studies have reported increasing prevalence of hypertension with urbanization; with it, access to processed food increases and fresh foods become less affordable and less available.

It is indisputable that hypertension has serious negative impacts on the microvascular and vascular systems of the body, especially the brain. There is a plethora of supportive evidence confirming the benefits of blood pressure management as a potential mechanism to reduce the risk of cognitive decline and dementia.

Sodium reduction is likely to benefit most people, especially those with hypertension and pre-hypertension. Because sodium is ubiquitous in the U.S. food supply, significant and large reductions in its intake are not easily attainable without any proactive and educated actions. At least 70% of sodium intake is derived from processed and restaurant foods.

If your high blood pressure remains elevated despite diet and lifestyle changes, consult your physicians for anti-hypertensive medication that has the least side-effects. Data pooled from six large observational studies suggest that anti-hypertensive medications may lower the risk of Alzheimer's disease and other forms of dementia. The review was published in Lancet Neurology in 2019.

The studies involved more than 31,000 participants older than 55, with

Follow-ups ranging from seven to twenty-two years. Among
the 15,537
Participants with the diagnosis of hypertension, those using
prescriptions
Had a 12% reduced risk for dementia and 16% reduced risk
of developing
Alzheimer's disease. The 15,553 participants with normal
blood pressure
Had the same risk for dementia as those who controlled
their blood
Pressure with medications. The type of medicines prescribed
in these
Studies made no difference.

Nowadays, many people, young and old, tend to rely too
much on the
Prescription medications, a temporary quick fix to control
their elevated
Blood pressure, instead of paying attention to their diets and
lifestyle for the
Long term benefits. After all, blood pressure prescriptions
do come with
Many adverse reactions (or side effects), affecting different
parts of the
Body including the mind.

In general, normal blood pressure is harder to maintain if
one is overweight,
Obese, or physically inactive. Hypertension is a major risk
factor for
Premature death, heart disease and stroke; and stroke is a
co-morbidity in up
30% of Alzheimer's patients, and it can be even higher.
Stroke undoubtedly
Can complicate and accelerate the progression of Alzheimer's
disease.

13. Keeping your blood sugar within the normal limits. Diabetes is so prevalent in the world, not just in the U.S., and many people don't even know that they are diabetic or pre-diabetic. Today, the average American consumes about 80 pounds of added sugar annually, or more than 23 teaspoons of added sugar daily. Ironically, experiments have demonstrated that an injection of sugar into the blood stream stimulates the same pleasure centers of the brain that respond to heroin and cocaine.

Poor control of blood sugar is the hallmark of diabetes mellitus. Excess glucose reacts with proteins to form Advanced Glycation End-products (or AGEs), which are actually oxidation products, blocking normal functioning and altering the structures of proteins. Studies have shown that the glycated hemoglobin becomes sticky when there is too much sugar in the blood, resulting in the production of AGEs. When AGEs form in the brain, the sticky damaged neurons can no longer transmit impulses effectively, preventing accesses to long- and short-term memories and thus increasing the risk of Alzheimer's disease. Please be reminded that almost any molecules in the body can suffer the same fate.

Like the amyloids, they are free radical amplifiers, formed by free radicals which exert their toxic effects by producing more free radicals resulting in oxidation stress and inflammation. One of the diabetic complications is atherosclerosis, which are harmful lesions in the micro-vasculature; it obviously reduces oxygen and nutrients to the eyes, heart, kidneys and the brain. Hypoglycemia occurs in uncontrolled and poorly controlled diabetes; these hypoglycemic episodes are stressful to the brain. That is why, diabetes in itself, is linked to a fourfold increased risk for Alzheimer's disease, according to many studies.

Sugar, by itself, is a major culprit in many health problems; elevated level of blood sugar is a significant contributing factor for the development of Alzheimer's. Insulin resistance is common among the older people, as is the loss of muscle mass, sarcopenia. But you can improve both undesirable conditions and decrease blood glucose levels by regular physical activities. By staying active such as walking, you stimulate the body to produce new mitochondria --- mitochondrial biogenesis, which improves the expression of signaling molecules to enhance memory and learning.

Patients with diabetes are at risk for early-onset dementia and mortality, especially among the middle-age group, according to researchers in Australia. The researchers at Curtin University conducted a retrospective study utilizing Western Australian hospital in-patients, mental health out-patient and death records to compare the age of dementia onset and survival outcomes among dementia patients with and without pre-existing diabetes. According to the findings, dementia onset occurred at an average of 2.2 years and death 2.6 years earlier in patients with diabetes when compared with patients without diabetes.

The public health significance of a 2.2 year age difference may seem modest and small, yet it has been estimated that any intervention including preemptive strategy as elucidated in this book capable of delaying the onset of Alzheimer's disease by two years would certainly reduce the projected tripling or quadrupling of Alzheimer's disease prevalence by year 2050 by at least 20%. These significant and meaningful findings have major implications for estimating the future Alzheimer's burden due to diabetes as well as clinical impacts for affected patients and their families.

It has become clearer and clearer that there is an association between dementia and diabetes, and after all, the brain is one of the end organs impacted by diabetes. If there are chronically high levels of blood glucose that are not controlled, it can adversely affect the brain as it does other areas of the body.

The importance of the linkage between type-2 diabetes and Alzheimer's disease dementia is perhaps best described by the term "type-3 diabetes", referring to some patients who develop Alzheimer's disease dementia as a result of diabetes-related damage and degeneration. In the Rotterdam study, meta-analytic data have demonstrated a significantly increased risk for Alzheimer's disease dementia among individuals with type-2 diabetes, up to 50% greater; and the heightened risk is even higher in people who were treated with insulin.

Logically, a low-carbohydrate is an effective and one of the healthy ways to help stem the tide of memory loss and cognitive decline. The percentage of carbohydrate in relation to fats and proteins must be individualized; but it is undeniable the modern American diet is characterized by excessive consumption of carbohydrates. Very few people will argue that our modern American diet is generally lower in phytonutrients and antioxidant-rich dark, leafy green vegetables and colorful fruits than the diet our robust ancestors consumed.

People with Alzheimer's should be more selective in eating fruits, ideally in the category of low to medium glycemic indexes to prevent spikes in blood sugar, hyperglycemia and hyper-insulinemia; they are both major risk factors of Alzheimer's disease.

Most consumers wrongly believe that artificial sweeteners are safe AND healthy, and good for weight loss because they do not have calories or very few calories. More and more scientific studies have discovered a host of harmful and unhealthy effects they have on the body, from obesity to the risk of certain cancers. Research has shown that artificial sweeteners do affect the blood levels of insulin resulting in hyper-insulinemia, because simply having a sweet sensation in your mouth is enough to stimulate the pancreas to secrete insulin with the expectation. The most insidious thing about the artificial sweeteners is that they might actually induce the cravings for additional sweet foods. So, for your general long-term health, it is best to avoid the artificial sweeteners altogether.

Excess insulin and beta amyloid protein fragments are both degraded and cleared by the Insulin Degrading Enzyme (IDE) in a normal equilibrium. But, when hyper-insulinemia becomes chronic, the IDE will prioritize to clear the insulin, allowing the beta amyloid to accumulate. Research has shown that when blood insulin levels are low, such as a low carbohydrate diet, the Insulin Degrading Enzyme is able to focus on degrading and clearing of beta amyloid proteins. In other words, a low-carbohydrate diet can be protective against Alzheimer's disease.

14. Learning Tai Chi if you can. This is an ancient Chinese exercise and practice, involves slow, focused, fluid movements along with rhythmic deep breathing. There are different styles of Tai Chi with different postures. Tai Chi, which is widely practiced daily in many public parks in China, is believed to open all the meridians and balance the practicing person's "qi". Many studies have shown and supported its beneficial effects on the physiology, psychology and kinesiology of the human body.

Tai Chi is an exercise of the mind and body to activate the neuro-muscular pathways to improve and enhance balance. Like walking and other aerobic exercise, it can stimulate your sensory and motor cortex, maintaining the brain's balance system. The U.S. National Council on Aging recognizes 14 programs for fall prevention, and Tai Chi is considered one of the most effective. Some studies have found that Tai Chi can help not only with balance, it can also reduce the incidence of falls, and enhance the quality of life for people with neuro-degenerative diseases such as Alzheimer's, Parkinson's disease and stroke.

In the U.S., more than one in four adults age 65 or older fall every year, resulting in many premature deaths in this age group. And more than 95% of hip fractures are the result of a fall. An injury or fracture due to a fall can set one's well-being back, adversely affecting the health of an older adult, especially one with Alzheimer's, with serious consequences. It is not just about learning the different Tai Chi moves as an exercise, it is also learning about the risks of falling and how to manage them with controlled movements.

For individuals in the early stages of Alzheimer's disease, they remain relatively active with intact mobility, they definitely can benefit from Tai Chi. Be sure that you understand your abilities and moderate your practice accordingly. When in doubt, consult your physician or a neurologist. One can do Tai Chi in a chair or standing independently.

The special exercise of Tai Chi requires concentration on the motor movements while stimulating the brain's balance system. Furthermore, Tai Chi has a meditation aspect, which is effective in reducing the levels of stress and anxiety; it can help preserve and strengthen memory and the hippocampal neurons according to some recent studies. What a graceful, elegant and healthy way to explore your personal space!

15. Getting adequate sleep. In the U.S., sleep deprivation is common even though most people do not realize it, or simply ignore it, unaware of the potential adverse and negative impact on our health and general well-being. Researchers have shown that chronic sleep deprivation causes increased

deposition of beta-amyloid plaques in the brain, thus raising the risk of Alzheimer's.

We all need adequate quality sleep, which allows the brain to rest and re-set. This "down time" is necessary so that neurotoxic and metabolic wastes can be eliminated optimally. Older people in general are light sleepers because they spend less time in the deep stages of sleep cycle. Getting a restful night's sleep for them is often complicated by some physical ailments, aches and pains. It must be pointed out that during deep sleep, also known as rapid eye movement (REM) sleep, the body including the brain heals and recharges itself.

General sleep hygiene should be followed including going to bed and getting up about the same time, and avoidance of stimulants like coffee and sea. No alcohol or cigarettes because they are absolutely harmful and inappropriate for people with Alzheimer's. Some medications can cause sleeping problems due to side-effects; you or caregiver should check with the prescribers and to see if the medications are necessary. It is my personal opinion that the less the medications for the Alzheimer's suffers, the less the complications.

Eating two to three hours before bed-time is not a good idea, especially salty, fried and fatty foods. As soon as you take the first bite, your digestive system kicks into action, and the body releases histamine which stimulates the production of acid to travel to the stomach to break down your food, Histamines may keep you awake. Too much salt can make you get up to go to bathroom more frequently. Night-time urination is or can be a real problem for many elderly people.

Melatonin can help some people get better sleep. Melatonin is converted from serotonin via the enzyme, methyltransferase inside the pineal gland. With age, there is a gradual decline of melatonin production. Its levels are normally higher at night time and lower during the day. With less melatonin for older people at night, thus they seem to suffer from insomnia more than young people.

Melatonin is known to be a free-radical scavenger, and therefore an antioxidant with many other health benefits including enhancement of the immune system and decrease in the rate of neuro-degeneration. Many studies have demonstrated the antioxidant property of melatonin and it may be neuroprotective and beneficial for Alzheimer's suffers. Taken orally, it is easily absorbed and quickly boosts its blood level. Some research have found that melatonin promotes the activities of the antioxidant enzymes, SOD and catalase, thus reducing or preventing neuronal apoptosis.

A recent study has found that older people who are prescribed a device to treat Obstructive Sleep Apnea (OSA) may have a lower risk of developing Alzheimer's disease and dementia. Researchers at Michigan Medicine's Sleep Disorders Center looked at 53,321 Medicare recipients over age 65 who had been diagnosed with OSA. This retrospective study by the medical scientists noted that people who used positive airway pressure devices (also known as CPAP) as prescribed were less likely to be diagnosed with dementia or Alzheimer's disease in the next three years than people who did not use CPAP. The findings of the study showed positive airway pressure (PAP) therapy was associated with lower odds for a diagnosis of incident Alzheimer's disease and also lower odds of mild cognitive impairment (MCI).

There is no doubt that chronic sleep deprivation is bad for mental health and there is such a profound, significant impact on cognition. Recent research, which followed about 8,000 people in their early 50s for a period of 25 years; those participants who slept less than 6 hours a night are

30% more likely to develop dementia later on in life usually starting in their 70s.

This increased dementia risk is independent of sociodemographic, behavioral
Cardiometabolic and mental health factors. In other words, chronic sleep
Deprivation in mid-life is associated with increased risk of late-onset dementia.
Short sleep is common nowadays, and its link to the
Increased risk of Dementia after mid-life is real and can be significant and
Important at a societal level.

16. Enjoy your coffee in moderation without sugar or cream. Coffee beans were first discovered by Ethiopia, an African nation many years ago; coffee has become the most common and prevalent beverage in the U.S. today. Coffee beans are an excellent source of antioxidants; researchers from the University of Scranton in Pennsylvania have found that coffee is a top-ranking winner of antioxidants. Coffee beans also contain many vitamins and minerals, such as riboflavin, pantothenic acid, niacin, thiamine, folic acid zinc, potassium, manganese and magnesium.

Several recent studies have shown that coffee drinking can improve cognitive functions such as alertness and focusing for Alzheimer's patients, in addition to the claim that consumption of coffee is associated with decreased risk of cancers of cancers of colon, breast and prostate. One study published in the European Journal of Neurology found a link between caffeine in coffee and protection against denervation of the brain in the early stages of Alzheimer's disease.

In the Nurses' Health Study of 83,000 women, researchers tracked their coffee drinking for 24 years; they discovered that women, who drank 2 to 3 cups of coffee a day without sugar, decreased their risk of stroke by 19%. Women who did not smoke in the study realized and reported even greater benefits. A decrease if the risk of stroke means a reduced risk for the development of Alzheimer's.

Other researchers have shown and confirmed that coffee heightens alertness and attentiveness, and improves mental performance and short-term memory. However, too many coffee drinkers tend to add sugar or artificial sweeteners; unfortunately, this added mixture nullify most of the health benefits of drinking coffee.

For individuals with Alzheimer's disease, having one to two cups of black coffee during the day should be health-promoting and beneficial, unless one has certain heart problems such as symptomatic or unstable tachy-arrhythmia such as atrial fibrillation.

17. Drinking green tea instead of sodas and other sugary beverages. Green tea is loaded with antioxidants and nutrients to help improve your well-being, both physical and mental. It has less caffeine than coffee. The beneficent compound in green tea is epigallocatechin 3-gallate (EGCG); and according to studies by researchers at Northwest A and F University in Yangling, China, EGCG can help lower insulin resistance, and improve memory impairment. The insulin functions better in the Central Nervous System with EGCG, suggesting that drinking green tea has a neuroprotective effect on the brain.

Catechins can be found in green tea, red wine and dark chocolate, but most of the studies have been from green tea. EGCG is a powerful antioxidant with anti-inflammatory and metal chelating abilities, thus, offering a neuroprotective effect on the brain.

18. Considering prophylactic therapy with low-dose aspirin. Both aspirin and non-steroidal anti-inflammatory drugs (NSAIDs) have anti- inflammatory properties; many people, especially the geriatric group, receive prescriptions for NSAIDs or simply buy them over-the-counter for their aches and pains and stiffness such as osteoarthritis.

Aspirin at a low dose of 81mg daily is recommended by many cardiologists to prevent blood clots that can cause heart attack and stroke. Several epidemiological studies have found that patients who were prescribed aspirin or NSAIDs for a number of years to control rheumatic or arthritic pain have less than half the risk of dementia.

Low dose aspirin could stimulate lysosomes to release their enzymes capable of breaking down the molecules from the beta-amyloid plaques. The findings have yet to be replicated in humans; but some experts are dubious and concerned because the long-term use of aspirin, even at low dose, can increase the risk of intra-cerebral hemorrhage in patients with Alzheimer's disease.

The concerns of potential hemorrhages, either in the brain or in the gastrointestinal tract are real and can be life-threatening with the long-term usage of NSAIDs and/or low-dose aspirin. The prophylactic therapy with daily low-dose aspirin must be individualized considering the benefit-risk ratio and the advice of your physician. One must exercise extreme care when considering the concomitant use of ASA for patients taking a direct oral anticoagulant (DOAC) for atrial fibrillation and/or venous thromboembolism due to increased risk of bleeding with uncertain and questionable therapeutic benefit.

19. Pursuit of new learning and education. Some of the remarkable reductions in the risk of developing Alzheimer's disease have been linked to higher levels of education --- with

each year of schooling beyond elementary levels considerably increasing the overall benefits. Furthermore, intellectual activities and late-life learning are well known and proven by researchers to offer protection from Alzheimer's disease and dementia.

In 2017, a group of European researchers studied the data of more than 55,000 people and found that the risk of dementia dropped with each completed year of formal education. Advances in education with mentally enriched environments, coupled with improvements in health care and living conditions could explain their reduced rates of Alzheimer's and dementia.

Mental challenge and enrichment of the surroundings, according to research, stimulate the development of new neurons and neural connections to compensate for any losses in cognitive capacity that would otherwise affect daily living adversely.

Education, in general, can also help individuals regardless of age to learn how to be more flexible and resourceful with their existing skills and knowledge. It is convincing and encouraging to know that education is a protective factor for Alzheimer's disease due to the "expanded brain reserve" from intellectual stimulation and enrichment. This is not to say that if you do not have higher education beyond elementary levels for some reasons in your life, you are doomed to get and suffer from Alzheimer's and dementia.

Neuroscientific studies have shown that an enriched environment and more things to learn and do can enhance the brain's general functioning and make a person "smarter". In fact, the enhanced activities of brain functions can be measured by functional magnetic resonance imaging (fMRI).

There are many things one can do and pursue in the learning processes to stimulate brain activities, leading to more active and more abundant dendritic branches and axonal terminals --- arborization. Higher levels of neuronal arborization produce a larger brain reserve. Higher education such as undergraduate college and graduate school is not the only route available for you to minimize the risk of Alzheimer's and to build up your resistance against this horrible disease.

Here are some suggestions:

- Learning a new language
- Learning to play a new musical instrument
- Learning a new skill or craft
- Reading a book and looking up the dictionary for the new vocabularies
- Reading a book to your children (social interactions)
- Playing non-violent video games and grabbing that joystick. Studies have found that this stimulates the parts of the brain that control movements, memory, planning and fine motor skills.
- Doing numbers and word puzzles. Games and puzzles are a great way to maintain your cognitive edge, according to studies by neuroscientists. They are also a fun way to spend time with the people you love and to bond with family and friends. They also promote social interaction, and are surely a wonderful pastime.
- Playing chess, cards, or mahjong (Mahjong is a Chinese or Asian game with small regular tiles shuffled and played on a Mahjong table. The number of players is usually four, but occasionally the game can be played with three people. The shuffling movements involve the arms, shoulders and neck, constituting a good exercise at a leisure pace.)
- Watching TV news or history/discovery channels, but not being a couch potato and avoid prolonged sitting.

- Signing up for a class at a community college, credit or non-credit, finding yourself in an intellectually stimulating surroundings with social interactions.
- Visiting a museum with friends or family.

Even though limited schooling may be a negative factor in terms of neuroprotection against Alzheimer's disease and dementia, it is your choice and within your power to overcome the pre-existing limitations and disadvantage and invest in your future for optimal brain health. And to enhance your brain reserve and increase your resistance against neuro-degenerative diseases like Alzheimer's.

The adult brains do make new neurons --- adult neuro-genesis when given the right, promoting and stimulating environments. Many recent studies in neuroscience have demonstrated the neurogenesis in the brain, including the hippocampus is possible and enhanced by new learning, new experiences, exercise, estrogen and environmental enrichment. Neuroplasticity and the ability of neuronal arborization of the brain make it possible to achieve neuroprotection against mental decline, to slow down or halt the progression of Alzheimer's, and even to reverse its course.

Learning something new with long term enrichment has an immense positive effect on promoting neurogenesis in an aging brain, as researchers have demonstrated. Simple re-doing already known or already-mastered skills cannot achieve neurogenesis, but challenging mental activities will increase and bolster survival of hippocampal neurons.

Many more studies suggest that people with more education seem better protected from mental decline, and the most likely and accepted explanation is that years of education has created a "brain reserve", also known as a "cognitive reserve, or "extra smartness", which can compensate or be called upon as the brain declines or degenerates.

Not all activities are equal in terms of brain enrichments, even though some activity or stimulation is better than none. For example, studying to play a musical instrument and dancing are associated with lower risk of dementia based on some neuroscientific research. In dancing, it requires learning new moves and rhythms, and is both physically and mentally challenging including concentration.

As we know, with all the scientific evidences, Alzheimer's disease is associated with the loss of brain cells, the neurons. Another striking feature of this multi-dimensional illness is the "use it or lose it "phenomena" like the musculoskeletal system of the body. It is a well-known principle in physiology that any part of the body that falls into disuse will begin to atrophy and wither away.

It is indisputable that late-life learning and intellectual activities offer protection from Alzheimer's disease and dementia. It seems almost as if Nature says "we know you are not physically strong enough to contribute to your community as a work-horse at this juncture of life, but we still value your wisdom and intellect. If you are not using and exercising your brain, then maybe it is time to bow out".

20. Staying socially connected is important for mental health. Many psycho-social studies have shown that social connections including interactions with family and friends reduce the risk of death from coronary heart disease, strokes and chronic illnesses such as Alzheimer's disease.

In the U.S., at least one in ten Americans live alone, and many are at risk for loneliness. Many of these lonely individuals are older, and the trend will continue because the geriatric population is the fastest growing segment of the world. Loneliness is "a disease of disconnection" which keeps you emotionally and socially isolated. Being isolated and lonely is very different from self-imposed, spiritual solitude as practiced by some religious groups such as the Tibetan or Buddhist monk. Solitude improves introspection and mental health, and enhances serenity and inner peace including equanimity.

Psychosocial researches have further shown that lonely people experience more insomnia, more depression, more susceptible to infections and less effective immune system. Lonely people face greater risk of premature death from all illnesses. People who have mutually caring interpersonal relationships enjoy increased sense of well-being and mental health, display greater emotional resilience, and live longer and happier lives.

During the Corona COVID-19 pandemic, isolation and social disconnection caused an increase of "brain fog" with poor cognitive function and poor memory, as admitted by many people under lock-down. The brain fog is further made worse with uncertainty and anxiety. Researchers of neurology and neurosurgery department at Duke University have shown that loneliness can change the neurochemistry of the brain. Loneliness is associated with reductions in brain-derived neurotrophic factor, BDNF, a protein important for neuronal health, cognition and memory.

A study in JAMA Psychiatry in 2016 found that older adults who have normal cognitive function but who are lonely showed more amyloid deposits in their brains on PET scans than their peers who are not lonely.

Physical touch is an important part of social connections and interactions; it includes hugging, handshaking and caressing. Haptics or the sense of physical touch is one of humanity's most basic ways of connecting and communicating.

Researchers have demonstrated that touching activates the cutaneous-visceral and viscero-cutaneous reflexes, that is, electrical connections between the internal organs and the skin.

Physical touch is primordial, being the first of our senses to develop; touching and being touched are essential for a healthy life. It can be a powerful, non-verbal communication, particularly for someone suffering from Alzheimer's disease. While personal touch during social interaction is a wonderful way to convey our feelings, but we have other channels for touching each other besides the skin. We connect with each other through all of our senses, with our eyes, our ears, our noses, our tongues, our bodies and minds.

Connectedness and nurturing are important for brain stimulation and mental health. Each of us came to this world through the body of another being. Every person was once part of his or her mother, connected to her body and contained and nurtured within it. We all bear the sign of that wonderful and blessed connection --- the umbilicus (navel or belly button). It is a sign of where we came from, and a membership card in the human club.

Social connectedness and interactions are critical and important for the Alzheimer's patients, especially in the early stages; find an organization to volunteer to help, if physically able, or walking in the park with your loved ones instead of marinating in negative thoughts. It is also crucial for the caregivers to stay socially connected. It is clear with convincing data that loneliness can have detrimental effects on overall health, especially on the brain, and lonely people have a higher risk of dementia.

The cerebral cortices of young rats reared in stimulating surroundings are packed with more neurons, synapses and dendrites than are found in rats kept in isolation, according to some studies. Certain of these studies specifically revealed increased number of neurons in the dentate gyrus of the hippocampus when adult rats and mice are housed with environmental stimulations. It is clear and convincing that staying socially connected can decrease your risk for development of Alzheimer's disease and make you more resistant to its relentless progression.

There is no doubt that staying socially engaged is crucial for brain health, especially pursuing social activities that are meaningful to you. I encourage you to find ways to be part of your local community --- if you love and enjoy their presence, consider volunteering or working in an animal shelter. If you like singing, join a local choir of a church. Or simply, just share activities with friends and family. According to a recent study published in the journal Neurology, researchers found that mentally stimulating activities that involve seeking and/or processing information, such as reading, letter writing, playing cards and doing puzzles, may delay the onset of dementia in older people. Many studies have shown that a cognitively active lifestyle in old age can delay the onset of dementia in Alzheimer's disease by as much as 5 years. These findings are definitely significant with important and far-reaching social impact.

21. Hormonal replacement therapy (HR) can be helpful and beneficial for some patients. Since there are more women suffering from Alzheimer's disease than men, most of the information here is directed toward post-menopausal women in terms of estrogen replacement therapy, ERT. There is some mention of testosterone therapy for older men when appropriate, and this is to be discussed later in this section.

According to one study of 427 post-menopausal women sponsored by the U.S. National Institute on AGING, researchers have found that ERT may reduce the risk of developing Alzheimer's. At the time of menopause, the neurons and circuits of the female brain that have depended on the estrogen for so long simply shrink and lose the vitality. Physiologically, estrogen is produced by the ovaries in large quantities about 24 months after birth of the infant girl --- called infantile puberty, marinating or inundating her young brain.

During puberty of the teenage years, the female brain will experience estrogen surges from the ovaries every month along with the increase of progesterone.

At menopause, the monthly hormonal waves with estrogen came to an abrupt stop; this physiological shock to her brain often leads to emotional turmoil for some women, commonly known as post-menopausal syndrome (PMS). Her first hot flash is a sign that her brain is starting to experience estrogen withdrawal.

Estrogen is known to affect the brain's levels of serotonin, dopamine, nor-epinephrine and acetylcholine --- neurotransmitters that can modulate mood and memory. It is logical and not surprising that peri- and post-menopausal changes in estrogen levels can influence different mental functions. Estrogen is more than just a "sex hormone". It is also used to regulate muscle and skeletal growth, maintain bone density, and help maintain the nervous system. So, the need for estrogen for the female brain which includes neurons, the neuro-circuits and the neuro-chemicals is not difficult to understand and appreciate, unless there is specific, absolute contra-indication for estrogen replacement therapy (ERT).

At Yale University, researchers found that post-menopausal women on ERT performed tests with brain patterns characteristic of younger women on the brain scans, while those without estrogen replacement therapy showed brain patterns typical of much older women.

Studies by neuroscientists at UCLA revealed that post-menopausal women on ERT were less depressed and performed better on cognitive tests. They also showed better working memory than did post-menopausal women who were not taking estrogen supplements.

Researchers at the University of Illinois found that the longer the post-menopausal women were on estrogen replacement therapy, the more the gray matter in the brain, i.e. corresponding increase in the brain cell volume.

Canadian researchers have studied the effects of estrogen on the brains of post-menopausal and post-hysterectomy women for over 25 years, and discovered the brain-preserving benefits of ERT in women who received ERT immediately after menopause and after their hysterectomies. For many of these women, ERT helps to stabilize their moods and improves their mental focus and memory. The neuroprotective effects of estrogen are remarkable and obvious.

From other studies of female rats given estrogen, it was observed that the number and length of the dendritic branches are increased in their hippocampus and frontal cortex.

Furthermore, researchers at the University of California, Irvine, had found that estrogen replacement therapy increased the efficiency of the mitochondria in the arteries of the brain, enhancing cerebral blood flow. This phenomenon helps to explain why pre-menopausal women have lower rates of stroke than post-menopausal women who are not on ERT. Thus, estrogen clearly can help the brain's blood flow stay strong for years into older age, reducing the risk of stroke and in turn the risk of Alzheimer's.

Post-menopausal women, for some reasons, have about three times higher risk than men for developing Alzheimer's disease. It is reasonable and clinically obvious to say that the low level or the lack of estrogen is a significant contributing factor to the elevated risk of strokes in post-menopausal women.

Many human studies have suggested that estrogen replacement therapy may be able to delay the symptoms of Alzheimer's disease and other dementia, and alleviate the aging of brain in older women, while modulating the physiological transition from menopause.

As for the ERT for post-menopausal women, there is a plethora of evidence that its benefits greatly outweigh any risk. Over a century ago, menopause was relatively rare because the average age of death for women was about 50 at that time. Many women today will likely live to be more than 100, a lot of years after menopause. The U.S. FDA recommends that women with menopausal symptoms take the lowest dose of estrogen for the shortest time possible. The decision for estrogen replacement therapy should be re-evaluated every twelve months with your physician with individualized treatment.

One of the most intriguing aspects regarding the epidemiology of Alzheimer's disease is the prevalence rate in women is approximately twice that in men, and this skewed sex ratio is specific for Alzheimer's, not for other forms of dementia. More and more research is suggesting that estrogen deficiency following menopause may contribute to the etiology of Alzheimer's disease in women.

Men tend to have shorter life spans than women and even though the gap of life span has narrowed as men are living longer, still at the age of 75 and older, there are significantly more women with Alzheimer's than men. As a summary for ERT, as demonstrated by many studies, estrogen promotes brain cell survival, neuronal growth and regeneration, including maintenance of brain function and protection against age-related mental decline.

Physiologically, testosterone levels in men peak around age 30 and going down gradually after that. This hormone in American men has been declining steadily over the past three decades as a trend, according to a study published in the prestigious Journal of Clinical Endocrinology and Metabolism. Despite the long-standing, somewhat questionable "bad boy" reputation, testosterone indeed has many health benefits. Here, just to name a few within the scope of this book:

- Testosterone keeps the brain of elderly men sharp and focused. According to studies by Dutch researchers, subjects with low levels of testosterone have increased risk of cognitive impairment and/or memory loss; some men with the cognitive and memory impairments developed Alzheimer's disease in the studies. A higher or normal level of testosterone improved their cognitive function and memory difficulty.

The heart is the organ with the highest concentration of testosterone receptors; the brain is second only to the heart in terms of abundance of testosterone receptors.

- Testosterone helps preserve muscle mass and, with exercise, reduce the risk of becoming frail as you age. The improved muscle mass and strength can help better neuro-muscular coordination, minimizing fall risk.

- Testosterone can help fight depression. Australian researchers have found that older men with low free testosterone levels have three times the risk of developing depression of men with high levels of free testosterone. As shown by many studies, depression is a known risk factor for Alzheimer's disease, even though many Alzheimer's patients are depressed for a number of reasons that we can all understand and sympathize with.

Anyway, hormonal replacement therapy, either with estrogen for post-menopausal and post-hysterectomy women, or testosterone for older men, must be individualized under the guidance and supervision of a physician, weighing benefits against risks, including the consideration for patients' quality of life.

Because we are dealing with the multi-dimensionality and unpredictability of a dementing illness, with different contributing and aggravating factors and possible multiple causes, it is unlikely, not meaning to sound pessimistic, that we will soon find a single drug that can eradicate Alzheimer's. Pharmaceutical research for Alzheimer's disease has been on-going for decades and should continue,

Do not hesitate to consult with knowledgeable health professionals if your spouse or loved one may have or show some early signs and symptoms of Alzheimer's with your suspicion, keen observation or instinctive 'gut feeling'. Time is of the essence. With Alzheimer's disease, there is generally a rather large window in the early stages of the illness for intervention; I call it the "redemptive period" which can extend up to eight years or longer before the late stage of the disease strikes if it happens despite all of your efforts and fighting strategies. The late stage of Alzheimer's is a horrendous, de-humanizing and heart-breaking time for both the victim and caregiver, and hopefully you and your loved one will be spared of the scourge!

- To conclude this section of fighting strategies to protect against Alzheimer's disease, some studies have found that many medicines, OTC or prescriptions, taken by many Americans for conditions such as depression, asthma and allergy may raise the risk for the development of Alzheimer's and dementia over time. The drugs involved in these studies are known as anti-cholinergics. Anticholinergics, either the sole component or a part of the drug, work by blocking a brain chemical called acetylcholine which is crucial and necessary for memory. The researchers in these studies looked at more than 100 over-the-counter and prescriptions that work in this way, including paroxetine used in many antidepressants, diphenhydramine found in many allergy medicines, dimenhydrinate in medications for motion sickness.

Researchers from the Indiana University School of Medicine found that older adults taking anticholinergics regularly were four times more likely to develop either mild cognitive impairment (MCI) or dementia than those not taking the medicines over time frame ranging from 6 months to about 8 years. As already known, some drugs used to treat Alzheimer's disease by increasing the amount of acetylcholine to improve memory. Another class of prescription drugs is the anti-psychotics, which are often prescribed to help manage agitation, anxiety, sleep problems. Some studies have shown that they can exacerbate dementia or increase the risk for dementia.

Other prescription medicines in addition to the anti-psychotics such as anti-depressants, anti-seizure drugs and opioid pain relievers all affect the brain and CNS with some documented adverse reactions. It is true that these medications including anticholinergics and over-the-counter medicines are approved by the U.S. Food and Drug administration and recognized as safe and effective when taken as instructed. However, research and other studies have shown a pretty strong association between these medications and higher risk of dementia, even though they cannot prove cause and effect.

It is impossible to calculate the extent of the association or linkage because these medications can be metabolized at different rates in different people, and they may have different effects on different people. If one has a diagnosis of Alzheimer's disease and/or dementia, it is prudent and careful to take those medicines, OTC or prescribed, only after serious discussion with your physician, and when it is absolutely necessary.

THE BENEFICENT
POWER OF WALKING

I deem it necessary to dedicate one entire chapter of this book to talk about walking as an exercise, and I just cannot emphasize enough about the importance of walking for all of us, especially for individuals suffering from Alzheimer's disease in their early stages. Walking is the exercise you can enjoy and benefit from even at ripe old age without causing damage to your joints. There is a lot of mention about walking 10,000 steps as a magic number; realistically, walking 10,000 steps a day seems unattainable for many people even with good intention. Research has shown that a daily walk around 7,500 steps regularly can give you very similar health benefits as 10,000 steps. Spending time or walking in green spaces, as many studies have demonstrated, is good for mental and physical health; of course, walking in rural areas by all means is healthier than the congested, inner cities with air pollution.

The vast, almost innumerable benefits of walking as an exercise on cardiovascular, physical and mental health are undisputed. Physical inactivity is the culprit of the disease process for many chronic, degenerative states. For the Alzheimer's sufferers in the early stages of the illness which can sometimes go for years, they have a "golden window of opportunity" to improve and maintain their physical and mental well-being while their muscle memories are essentially intact with locomotive abilities.

It is irrefutable that therapeutic intervention is likely to be most effective early on before extensive death of neurons. The most important and necessary thing for human survival, after oxygen, water, salt and food is exercise which includes walking. Human beings are meant to walk; we are bipedal, erect species with bodies designed for locomotion.

In the early stages of the late-onset Alzheimer's disease, the individuals are generally ambulatory, able to use and move their arms and legs, unless they are also suffering from debilitating co-morbidities. Of course, most elderly people in their late 60s and 70s are not being expected to be runners, but they can walk to satisfy the body's needs for aerobic exercises. Just walking 25 to 30 minutes a day, you will reap all the terrific health benefits, both for the body and mind. Furthermore, the frequency and duration of walking can be increased, if so desired, as long as the weather permitting and the caregivers available as companions.

Walking is a complex behavior and a very healthy bodily function, but many of us in our modern, digital world have taken it for granted or simply forget about it; they become sedentary in their lifestyle, night and day without realizing the serious consequences for their general health. The high cost of a sedentary lifestyle just became more evident with a new global study showing that inactivity drives I in 14 deaths. These findings, based on population data for 15 health outcomes across 168 countries, were published in March, 2021 in the British Journal of Sports Medicine.

Walking requires functional integration of a lot of sensory and motor interaction and experience; it activates the brain and the musculoskeletal system. One of the important components of walking is balancing. In order to maintain the body's balance unconsciously and effortlessly as it changes position and moves over somewhat uneven terrain in a gravitational field, the brain needs and interacts with different information. It relies partly on a mechanism in the inner ears responsible for sensory orientation in three- dimensional space. If this function of inner ear fails, you cannot maintain equilibrium.

Besides the ears, the brain also requires visual input of information from other senses to keep the walking person in balance: from the tactile receptors which let the brain know which part of the body is in contact with the ground, and from the proprioceptors in the muscles, tendons and joints that keep the brain continuously informed of the exact position of each part of the body in space. Dysfunction in any of these neural circuitries can lead to erratic movements and falling.

The cerebellum, located below the occipital lobes of the cerebrum, processes all of these sensory input to coordinate responses of muscles to the ever-changing requirements of ambulation. Research shows that exercise stimulates the sensory and motor cortex and maintains the brain's balance system. These functions begin to deteriorate gradually as we get older, making us prone to falling and becoming home-bound and bed-confined. Nothing accelerates the atrophy of the brain more than being immobilized in the same environment with little stimulation.

Normal walking involves movements of the limbs in cross-patterned fashion: the right leg and the left arm move forward at the same time, then the left leg and the right arm. Researchers believe that the cross-patterned movements seem to have a harmonizing influence on the Central Nervous System while generating electrical activities in the brain, and bolster normal development and optimal functioning of the human brain.

Researchers of observational studies believe that when the babies first start to crawl, their cross-patterned movements serve to stimulate optimal brain development. This coordinated movements of crawling may look regressive and odd for the grown-ups, especially for those who have difficulty walking, but it may be a good exercise for the brain. Some older adults may want to try crawling on a clean carpeted floor with the caregiver around, and have some good workout/exercise. Personally, I think there is nothing to lose in terms of physical and mental health, and everything to gain!

An eye-opening experiment was conducted by Swedish psychologist, Dr. Bengt Saltin, who had five volunteers for three weeks to assist him in the study of extended bed-rest on the body. The five young men in the experiment were physically fit, but at the end of the three weeks laying in beds, all of them showed a reduction in the aerobic capacity that equated with twenty years of aging. The experiment confirmed the paramount importance of bodily movements and exercise in maintaining and promoting good health and slowing the aging process.

Let us look at the numerous health benefits from regular walking 25 to 30 minutes a day, at least five days a week:

- Walking for stronger bones --- As we age, we lose the ability to absorb sufficient calcium into the body and the bones become thinner, leading to osteoporosis. Osteoporosis is a common cause of fractures among the elderly, hip fractures in particular. Statistically, hip fractures strike at least one out of three women and one out of six men. Walking stimulates the body's assimilation of calcium and other nutrients.

  A gradual exposure to the sunlight with walking could be a wonderful and natural way to increase calcium absorption into the body and bones to minimized and/or prevent osteoporosis. Studies have shown that walking increases bone mass (bone density), not only in the legs, but also the arms. It is so important to be vigilant and cautious to avoid accidental falls or any injury that can result in fractures, which will set you back with immobilization, potentially subjecting you to many health problems.

- Walking can help lowering the blood pressure --- the walking movements open up the capillaries in the muscle tissues by reducing the resistance to blood flow in the arterial beds, causing the blood pressure to drop. That's

  Why walking is highly recommended for people with hypertension among
  Other things. Many researchers have shown and agreed that that a normal

Blood pressure helps to lower the risk of heart disease, stroke
    and
Alzheimer's disease.

- Walking can help decrease swelling in the lower
  extremities --- the contractions and relaxations of the leg
  muscles during walking help mobilize and overcome the
  force of gravity. Thus, the blood pooling in the leg veins
  is pushed upward (proximally) against gravity by frequent
  contractions of muscles in the lower extremities.

  This also causes an equally effective flow within the
      lymphatic system and
  Decrease edema in the legs; this consequentially eliminates
      the swelling
  With the venous and lymphatic systems.

- Walking burns glucose and decreases insulin resistance. As
  one gets older, insulin sensitivity decreases; walking can help
  improve insulin sensitivity and lower blood glucose level. In
  other words, walking can improve management of diabetes;
  a well-controlled diabetic means lower risk for Alzheimer's
  disease because of decreased levels of insulinemia.

- Walking, like other exercises, stimulates the release of
  endorphins in the brain and help fight stress and depression.
  This leads to improved moods and better sleep, especially
  for the elderly.

- Walking improves circulation and the elasticity of the
  arteries, making the heart a more efficient pump, thus,
  improving cerebral circulation and providing more
  oxygen and nutrients to the brain. Optimal cerebral blood
  flow clearly can decrease the risk for the development of
  Alzheimer's disease and make you feel mentally sharper.

- Walking promotes the movements of the intestines, bolstering and enhancing peristalsis, thereby helping constipation, which is a common problem for the geriatric group. It is physiologically important to have efficient eliminations of metabolic wastes to maintain optimal functions of the body and the brain with hemostasis.

- Walking can help you lose weight --- walking is a really good form of exercise and it can help you reach your fitness and weight-loss goals. However, when it comes to weight loss workout strategies, walking is totally underrated. It is time to change that attitude and misconception. Not only can you lose weight by doing it, but the more you weigh, the easier it is going to be dropping pounds. Generally, it varies from person to person as to how much weight you can lose by walking routine.

There is no magic formula for how many steps, miles, or hours you must walk to lose the amount of weight that you want. If you have a sedentary desk job, a walk every evening after dinner may surprise you with real results. There are many talks about a baseline of 10,000 steps a day; It is best to do more than you are doing now.

It is important to get in the habit of walking every day. Just make it part of your daily routine – something you do without even thinking about it. The best way to shed pounds off is to challenge yourself with intervals – periods of faster walking if you are physically able to do so. Research found that interval walkers lose more weight than people who just go the same speed all the time. So, you will get more bang for your buck by increasing your walking pace at intervals.

Overweight and obesity can bring you brain problems besides many other health issues. According to one large recent study of more than 8,500 people over the age of 65 published in the Journal of Neurology, people who are obese in middle age with a Body Mass Index of 30 or above, are at almost four times greater risk of developing dementia such as Alzheimer's disease in later life than people of normal weight. Growing scientific evidence suggests that controlling your body weight and maintaining a healthy weight can really reduce your risk of dementia.

- Walking is known to decrease the amount of undesirable body fats and the levels of serum cholesterol with less deposits within the arterial walls, thus, reducing the occurrence of atherosclerosis. We know that atherosclerosis, indisputably, is a major risk for heart attack and stroke, and stroke is a contributing factor for up to 30 to 25% of Alzheimer's cases, according to the many findings at autopsies of Alzheimer's patients.

- Walking can help tone the respiratory system and increase the exchanges of oxygen and carbon dioxide. By age 65, the lungs lose as much as 40% of their capacity to utilize oxygen, this is partly due to the decreasing numbers of alveoli and corresponding capillaries of the lungs with aging.

- Walking and other mild exercises all lead to lower levels of oxidative stress, according to research. Reduced levels of oxidative stress in the body minimize the formation of beta-amyloid plaques.

However, vigorous exercise often causes considerable oxidative damage due to higher demand for energy; it is difficult to know at what point you begin to do more harm than good. It is generally accepted that it is more beneficial with more gentle/mild aerobic exercise, like walking and leisurely swimming.

- Walking can increase the release of brain derived neurotrophic factor (BDNF) a protective protein in the brain, and this is found to improve learning and memory, according to many studies. In a 2011 meta-analysis of 15 studies that followed more than 33,000 people for up to 12 years, physical activity including walking provided a buffer against cognitive decline and poor memory with its many other health benefits, both physically and mentally.

According to neuroscientific research, exercise stimulates the production and release of BDNF, a neuronal growth factor, which plays a crucial role in effecting neuroplasticity and cognitive function. Simply walking at a good pace has been shown to bolster the growth of new neurons; patients with Alzheimer's disease tend to have reduced BDNF levels compared to healthy, normal people.

• Walking, like other forms of exercise, is a powerful stimulator of "mitochondrial biogenesis". Studies have demonstrated that aerobic exercise can increase the number and size of mitochondria in muscles, allowing the muscles to become more efficient at extracting oxygen from the blood. Research further has shown that energy shortage in the brain due to dysfunctional mitochondria can increase the level of the precursor for formation of the bet-amyloid plaques.

• Walking, like other aerobic exercise or physical activities, can slow down the progress of age-related changes of the brain, i.e. decrease tissue losses in the cerebral cortex, hippocampus and the cerebral white matter. The amount of shrinkage from the aging process, if unchecked, is most dramatic in the hippocampus, as much as 30% according to some research.

Our bodies are made for movements and activities, whether you walk rapidly or slowly, it makes little difference in terms of health benefits.

- The nerve conduction time decreases with age due to demyelination. Research has shown that physical activity and aerobic exercise can retard such age-related changes and facilitate re-innervation of damaged nerves.

- When walking, it is good and healthy to look at distant objects because looking at the distance helps to relax the ciliary muscle and suspensory ligaments of the lens of the eyes. This can help to decrease the risk of age-related macular degeneration, which is a common cause of blindness among the older population.

While you are walking, enjoy the fresh air and nature, connecting with the nature spiritually. Many studies have shown that our spiritual connections improve the immune system and decrease depressive moods; this is beneficial for someone with Alzheimer's. Many people believe and many studies have shown that walking is nature's effective and inexpensive anti-depressant. Walking just 10 to 12 minutes a day can build and improve your self-confidence according to some psycho-social studies.

Movement is a natural function, and it should be maintained, if at all possible and as long as possible. Walking can help increase a sense of well-being and vitality. Walking undoubtedly can improve physical and mental health for anyone; the older generation needs it even more, especially for individuals who already have chronic diseases such as heart problems and Alzheimer's disease.

In the early stages of Alzheimer's, locomotion is usually possible because the muscle memories are relatively intact. The absence or lack of significant physical disruptions at this time period provides a crucial and considerable window of opportunity for intervention. Neuroscientific research has already demonstrated that physical activities, like walking, stimulate the sensory and motor cortex and maintain the balance system of the brain.

There are two ways we can maintain the overall, optimal function of our brain: one is by creating new neurons, and the other is by extending the life of existing neurons. Physical activities or exercises and learning something new work in complementary fashion: physical activities can help make new neurons and new learning can help prolong neurons' survival.

For Alzheimer's patients in their early stages, their walking pace and gait will improve with regular practice, perseverance, and support from the caregivers. Here are a few words of safety precaution:

- Never attempt to walk alone
- Making sure that the terrain is level and without any visual obstruction
- Avoid noisy and crowded surroundings to minimize distraction
- Looking for and picking a visual target
- Be familiar with the walking area so that you will not become a victim of crime
- Take some rest at intervals if needed, especially you are in the beginning of this endeavor

A recent study of cognitively impaired, older adults, which was published in the "Journal of Alzheimer's Disease" found that just 30 minutes of brisk walking improve cerebral blood flow, and enhance memory, and cognitive functions. Please be reminded that any exercise is good and beneficial, if it is within your power. Exercise is perhaps the closest thing we have to a miracle drug for brain health. Even if you don't do it all the time or on a regular basis. It is absolutely incontrovertible that the bodily movements of exercise can improve your cognitive performance and memory function, and more importantly, minimize and/or avoid the risk of dementia.

Squatting seems to be the one form of exercise which offers remarkable, considerable benefits for the body and the mind. It is more difficult and intense than walking, and it may not be doable for some people or Alzheimer's patients. However, squatting presents intermittent positive hemodynamic challenges for the brain, according to the research conducted at the UK's University of South Wales' Neurovascular Research Unit. The hippocampus, which is a crucial part of our brain for memory function and learning, tends to shrink with aging. The researchers demonstrated that squatting nourishes the brain, especially the hippocampus. Their findings should not be surprising because when you squat, you are using most of your body's major muscle groups together simultaneously below the chest.

So, squatting 3 to 5 minutes and 3 to 5 times a week may help you beat back Alzheimer's disease!

ALZHEIMER'S DISEASE AND THE CAREGIVER

Most of the patients with Alzheimer's disease are receiving their care at home from their family, either the spouse, a close relative, or adult children. A small number of them are placed in nursing homes, usually in their late stages. Some of these institutions may have special care units, or memory care units for the Alzheimer's patients, and some of them may be placed and cared for among the general nursing home residents at the long-term facilities.

The current estimate of people with Alzheimer's in the U.S. is about 5 million. By the year 2050, the number of patients suffering from Alzheimer's is expected to be doubled at least in the U.S., reaching close to 15 million; globally, this most common form of dementia will affect more than 130 million people according to the estimate by the World Health Organization. The number of caregivers will also rise considerably with millions of hours of unpaid care with much unspoken personal sacrifice and expenses and enormous costs to the society.

A caregiver in a home setting is unequivocally subject to tremendous stress sustained over a long period of time with your loved one's demands and uncertainty. Caring and managing for this chronic dementing illness with physical and mental disabilities, interjected by periodic, unpredictable medical emergencies or night-marish episodes, is extremely grueling, frustrating and sometimes frightening.

Taking care of your loved one with Alzheimer's disease at home is a totally uncharted territory and experience for many people. Among many other things, be sure that you are aware of and know the limits of the impaired person's abilities which can be dwindling slowly every day. For example, do not take his or her words that he or she can heat up suppers or get into the bath-tub by themselves. You must be observing and observant as the impaired person does or perform various tasks.

Sometimes, they don't know what is edible and what is not; or they may drink something toxic liquid or poison by mistake. So, you must exercise or use your anticipatory precaution around them. At home, typically most of the accidents and incidents happen in the kitchen and the bathroom. The confused and impaired person often spills water or beverage on the floor of kitchen or bathroom, and forget to wipe it up or clean it, making it easy and dangerous to slip and fall on a wet spot for both the caregiver and individual with Alzheimer's.

For instance, do not assume any competency of your impaired loved one around a pool, even if he or she has always been a good swimmer because he may lose the judgment or ability to handle himself or herself in the water. This holds the same truth for the water of the lake or river or ocean front such as beaches. Here is a fairly common but very dangerous situation: an impaired or confused person in a care may open the door and attempt to get out or disembark while the vehicle is moving. So, seat-belts must be properly used and all car doors must be locked at all times. Having a preemptive and preventive strategy is of paramount importance as a caregiver for someone with Alzheimer's; there is no doubt that this is stressful and exhausting for you, both physically and mentally.

In my personal experience with the family, when having dinner or eating together, whether at home or in a restaurant, the caregiver must keep in mind that the person with a dementing illness is impaired may begin to use the hands instead of silverwares due to problem with coordination sometimes. It is easier for you to adjust to the embarrassing messiness than to fight or criticize it, or to show annoyance and displeasure.

Keep in mind that you will live with and experience many unexpected incidents or episodes when taking care of someone with

Alzheimer's disease, and to you, they don't make any sense at all. These happenings can be very frustrating, irritating, embarrassing and exhausting, mounting up day after day, and understandably and certainly, it can wear you out even the most patient and loving caregiver. Unfortunately, expressing your anger and other negative feelings and emotions to the 'sick person' often will make the matter worse because the Alzheimer's disease, a dementing illness, makes it impossible for the impaired person to respond to your anger in a rational manner.

Despite the resilience of human beings and the steadfast devotion of the caregiver, our psychological/physiological balance can be pushed over the edge, becoming dysregulated and dysfunctional if it is taxed beyond its limits to adapt and respond. Short- and long-term plans and strategies should be developed for adapting to the unfortunate situations, otherwise, the pressures of daily living and coping can reach a point where the caregiver is constantly in a state of hyper-arousal, reacting constantly to the stressors 24/7 with tension, anger and irritability, eventually leading to the feelings of helplessness and hopelessness.

As a devoted caregiver for your loved one suffering from Alzheimer's disease, the challenges can be overwhelming, to say the least. Studies have shown that depression among caregivers is common, and once chronic depression sets in, it will lead to changes of the hormonal and immune systems, resulting in "break-down". This break-down is essentially a state of psychological exhaustion with loss of enthusiasm and drive for life. Sometimes, the deepening depression can reach a point of requiring hospitalization and medications for the caregivers.

Some studies found that the wounds of Alzheimer's caregivers took longer time to heal than those of a control group due to the compromised function of the immune system. Surprisingly, many of them continued to show decreased immune responses even years after their loved ones, the Alzheimer's patients, passed away. Indeed, the sustained stresses with chronic depression in caring for the Alzheimer's setting can age the immune system of the caregivers prematurely, making them vulnerable and susceptible to many, different illnesses.

Researchers in social science have observed that although it may be at times difficult to admit how they feel, Alzheimer's caregivers often experience over time anger or deep-seated resentment towards those they love and care for – I call it reactive ambiguity. The feelings of anger and frustration can conceal your pain and grief inside you at a deeper level.

Many caregivers may continue to feel frustrated and angry that the persons they whole-heartedly are taking care of are no longer the persons they used to be. Such slow-burning resentment, a subconscious emotion, may not be easy to acknowledge or accept at a conscious level because it is clearly and ironically in conflict with the caregivers' sense of love, devotion and duty. This conflicting predicament or 'reactive ambiguity' is very likely to impact the caregivers' health and potentially immense costs to our society, and this must be taken seriously!

Social supports, private, NGO and governmental, are very important and urgently needed, given the scope and profound complexity of this growing socio-medical problem, which is going to reach an epidemic proportion, if not already, with our ever-increasing geriatric population in the U.S. and worldwide, not including the large segment of caregivers also affected.

If you are taking care of your aging and ailing parent, spouse or other beloved older family member afflicted with this terrible disease, you most likely feel drained and stretched, both in time and energy, not including financial losses and expenses associated with Alzheimer's care. It is a formidable, long and painful journey for both the caregiver and the victim. The magnitude of what you are dealing with profoundly immense, overwhelming and daunting, to say the least, and much of it invisible.

The psychic toll is actually the heaviest and unfathomable. Being a caregiver to someone you dearly love with Alzheimer's disease, is and will be the most difficult and saddest thing ever done and encountered in your life. With so many roles you have to take on: you are your impaired, loved one's ally, protector, social organizer, comforter, cook, driver, prompter, initiator, financial manager, plus more with the ever-changing situations and unexpected, heart-rending episodes and occasional medical emergencies.

Both the caregiver and the patient experience despair and loneliness in parallel; it is very important for the caregiver to reach out for help. Here are some suggestions:

- There are many reasons for the caregiver to feel fatigued, and the continued care of a person with Alzheimer's can be extremely exhausting and emotionally draining. You must ensure that you have adequate sleep and rest, including occasional naps during the day. When you are rested with sufficient sleep, you will feel better and manage better.

- You are doing a very difficult, twenty-four-hour job coupled with multiple responsibilities and overlaid with many mixed emotions. So, you must take some quality time for yourself --- this is not being selfish. To have time away from the sick, impaired person, to have friends to enjoy things you like, and to share your problems with. This will help lessen the tension and pressure with some diversion.

- Find a hobby or continue your favorite one.

- Take a walk with someone if available. Of course, it is ideal and wonderful if you and your impaired loved one can walk together. Working out, talking to friends on the telephone, finding a refuge, or meditating in a quiet place for relaxation and spiritual support.

- It is normal emotion to grieve for your continued losses in your loved one suffering from Alzheimer's, but allow yourself to dream new dreams.

- Accept any offer of help from friends or family members; however, you need to provide some specific instruction and suggest specific things that can be done.

- Learn as much as possible about your loved one's conditions associated with Alzheimer's disease, and try to focus on his or her remaining abilities.

- Seek support and friendship from other caregivers because there is strength in knowing that you are not alone.

- Trust your instinct to make the right decision; consider adult day care when necessary for your loved one because you cannot do everything all the time.

- Singing familiar songs with your loved one who is impaired to certain extent, or turning on your favorite music radio station for both of you. Indeed, studies have revealed that singing, especially singing together improves mental and emotional well-being. These subjective improvements are accompanied by measurable physiological changes with increased levels of immunoglobulin A, enhancing the immune system. Studies with residents of nursing homes who sang together showed significant reductions in stress, anxiety and depression, compared with those residents who did not sing.

  In patients with dementia, both singing and listening to music alleviated some of their troubling symptoms, including depressive mood, aggressive and agitated behaviors. The beneficial effects of music and singing are so well-established that they form the basis of music therapy.

- Eating with your family and your loved one with Alzheimer's as often as possible. Research has shown consistently that health benefits of communal eating extend beyond merely eating in the company of others. It provides an opportunity for communications including conversation, story-telling, and re=connection, in addition to improved digestion.

  With the pace of modern life and hectic schedules, more and more people tend to eat alone at a hurried pace, with fewer meals at the table with family, except for special holidays. They eat in the cars, at the desks while working and in front of the TVs; multi-tasking and the lack of mindful eating have become a common phenomenon. In a 2015 study published in the journal Appetite, people, especially the older ones who eat alone tend to have a poor appetite with poor, unhealthy eating habits, leading to poor nutrition.

- Mixed and ambivalent feelings are common when taking care of someone with Alzheimer's disease and other dementing illness; these feelings include anger, grief, despair, guilt, discouragement, helplessness and hopelessness. When your coping skills are overwhelmed and things seeming to drift out of control, counseling can be a great help to you and your family struggling with providing constant care to your loved one with physical and mental impairments.

  Most people seeking counseling are not 'sick', 'crazy' or 'neurotic' or 'mental', they are 'normal' people who sometimes have difficulty coping with real problems. Such sources of help may come from your priest or pastor, an objective close friend, a social worker, a nurse, psychologist, or a physician. Don't be afraid to seek outside help and get yourself out of the circular thinking. Getting counseling is not a sign of weakness. With the heavy burden you carry in coping with and caring for the impaired person you love, you can use and garner all the help you can get, and this is not a reflection on your strength.

- Praying for spiritual inspiration and support. If you have a religious affiliation, join your organization regularly. The positive impact of faith in the lives of 80% of the world's population who are involved in organized religion is undeniable. Many studies have shown that faith give you a sense of meaning and purpose that can overcome incredible adversity.

Toward the end of this harrowing, ruthless journey of "loss", instead of remaining silent about the subject of dying and death, it will be less tormenting and less daunting to talk about it openly with caring family and friends, including the patient who may be able to express and convey their wishes, if not already disclosed. For some people, the role of faith will be central and significant at this juncture. The forlorn feeling of life is a cruel feature of Alzheimer's disease for both the caregivers and the patients, from the beginning to the end!

Recent studies have revealed that even in patients severely affected by Alzheimer's disease in its late stages, their sense of identity is less compromised than might expect. Tape recordings of their speeches by researchers show that if their long pauses between utterances are removed, the listener will realize that the patients are more coherent than they appear to be. Care givers must learn to listen with greater patients and tolerance and attention, allowing more time for the patients to respond.

Realistically, nobody really knows what a person with Alzheimer's disease can and cannot comprehend, or what is going on inside his or her head. Your presence including others serves as an anchor for the Alzheimer's sufferers who is experiencing a disappearing world, desolate and fearful. In the presence of others, remember to include the impaired person in the conversation with physical touch and visual contacts. Sadly, people tend to cut the patient out of conversation unconsciously, as if the patient were not present. The caregivers need to keep letting go of expectations and be ready with whatever is happening with your steadfast, unchanging love.

Some special notes for the caregivers:

For scientific measurements and more precise understanding of Alzheimer's disease's trajectory, there are different stages and substages of this chronic illness for practical and simple purposes, early stage of Alzheimer's generally includes stages 1 to 3 or 4 when the Alzheimer's suffers are still ambulatory with intact muscle memories. With further impairments including the working memory, the illness progresses and advances to middle and late stages.

With the slow and gradual progression of the disease, the human awareness of the deficits can last for many years. We can roughly divide this dementing illness from the perspectives of awareness into two phases, even though there is no clear-cut separation: the awareness phase and the post-awareness phase. For quite some period of time, the Alzheimer's sufferer is usually aware that something is not quite right. Then, at a certain point, usually years into the illness, he or she no longer knows due to the loss of awareness.

The clinical stages such as early, middle and late stages are not to be confused with the Braak staging which refers to the spread of the Tau tangles in different regions of the brain. Pathologically, Braak stages one and two demonstrate the tangles in the entorhinal cortex, a region located near the base of the skull that is important for memory. Braak stages 3 and 4 show the tangles spreading higher and deep into the brain and involving the hippocampus and surrounding tissues. When the Tau tangles invade the neo-cortex, Braak stages 5 and 6 are reached.

Finding support group is important and beneficial for both the caregiver and patient from the early stage on. The Alzheimer's Association can provide helpful information and guidance for the patient and family members. As a caregiver, you are not alone, and together you can share your thoughts and feelings, learning and working on coping mechanisms and skills, and building strength in unity to face down this disease.

The support group can also help dealing with the denial and acceptance predicaments, confronting the uncomfortable truth head-on in the grieving process. With each passing year, the caregiver can find support and comfort in the transition from the early stages to the late stages with inner peace and shared knowledge, and meanings and purpose of life. The Alzheimer's support group can also be attended by close friends and adult children who may find it difficult to express their feelings. As the primary caregiver, you want to encourage them to share their thoughts and feelings to help dealing with this long ordeal. Sometimes we need to grieve together, and the tears and mutual connections will give all of you relief.

During the early stages of Alzheimer's disease, including the pre-clinical period, the faculty of ambulation is essentially unscathed and intact; this 'blessing' enables the afflicted individuals with some independence. But, because of their impaired cognitive ability and memory which can vary from person to person, this physical independence can be dangerous if not managed carefully with preemption and anticipation by the caregivers.

Wandering, a purposeless and aimless moving around or walking by the victim is a common problem and a serious challenge for the caregiver, family members and friends. The Alzheimer's patient cannot make sense out of what he or she sees and hears; and most of their behaviors are not under their control. As already described, people with dementia are often unaware of the extent of their impairment.

Oftentimes, just walking to the neighborhood store nearby, the Alzheimer's patient can become disoriented and completely lost just making a wrong turn. Or he or she may go shopping with you, lose sight of you and get lost trying to find you. Wandering can become more frequent when moving to a new home or in a new environment. They can wander onto busy streets, posing considerable dangers.

You, as a caregiver, must understand that the impaired person may no longer have the judgment such as wandering in front of a moving vehicle or stepping over the edge of a swimming pool. Sometimes the wandering person can become agitated, confused and anxious; situations like this requires your gentle reassurance, your calmness and understanding with steadfast love and devotion.

There are devices available to restrain an impaired person in a chair or bed if wandering becomes out of control with frequent problem and danger. This is not an easy decision to use physical restraint on the person you love and care for; it is best to make the decision jointly with healthcare professionals who know the patient and with family members who also help provide care to avoid misunderstanding and uneasy feelings. It is also a good idea for the caregivers to visit local medical supply stores to learn and look at what kind of restraint is available such as Posey and Gerichairs and so on. The Alzheimer's patients should wear some form of medical IDs like a bracelet with name and phone number, and a simple label: Alzheimer/Memory impaired.

Communication with an Alzheimer's patient is not easy, and this is truly an under-statement. Communications can be verbal or non-verbal, or a combination of both. The limitations in the impaired person's ability to communicate and express can be frustrating and confusing for both the patient and the caregiver. For example, the impaired person may burst into tears or simply walk away in anger when he or she is not understood. Sometimes, the impaired person may use curse words, even if they have never used such language before.

The impaired person, sometimes, may not be able to communicate the whole thought but can only express a few words about the thought. In some situations, the impaired individual may ramble on fluently, and it seems as if he or she is talking a lot in that moment yet making very little sense to the listeners. It is advisable and important for the caregiver to listen carefully and attentively; it is possible to understand what the impaired person is saying if you know the context.

Alzheimer's patients will communicate better when they are relaxed, so caregivers must appear relaxed and create a calm environment. You need to utilize simple questions when inquiring about the impaired person's needs; they may be able to utter a few words in response, or shake or nod their heads. In reference to a body part, you need to point to it in addition to naming it. Alzheimer's sufferers have difficulty comprehending or understanding what other people tell them. This can present a problem, being misinterpreted as "uncooperative behavior". In some cases, some Alzheimer's patients can have trouble understanding written information even when they can read letters or newspapers. For instance, when you hand the impaired person the written instruction "Turn your head to the right", he or she does not follow to do it even though they can read the written instruction. This can be irritating and infuriating until you realize that reading and understanding are two different skills.

Thus, do not assume that your loved one with Alzheimer's can understand and act upon your written messages because he or she can hear and read. The problem with communication can become worse on the telephone, it is not due to inattentiveness or willfulness, it is because the impaired person cannot make sense out of the words heard. A caregiver must speak slowly and clearly, using short words and simple sentences. Minimize, or better yet, eliminate distracting noises or activities. Caregivers should avoid high pitch of your voice because the impaired listener may interpret it as anger. Furthermore, caregivers ask only one short or simple question at a time, and repeat it as necessary.

It is not easy or pleasant to remind yourself that you are living with and taking care of your loved one who is suffering from Alzheimer's. Your non-verbal communications are very important with profoundly significant impact. Be calm, pleasant and supportive. Smiling and gentle touching can mean a great deal to the impaired person who feels isolated. Watch for body language and look directly at him or her with eye contacts.

Do not hesitate to use physical ways of expressing affection such as holding hands, hugging, putting an arm around his or her waist, light kissing on the face or lips, or just sitting close together. Even a person is mentally impaired, he or she stills needs and enjoys and appreciates affection, and the positive effects are mutual!

In the long years of taking care of an ALZHEIMER'S patient, all caregivers need rest and relaxation (R and R). Moreover, all caregivers will experience changes or addition of roles and responsibility (another R and R). The caregivers, woefully, will find very limited or finite time for rest and relaxation, even though it is crucial and important for their total well-being to nurture themselves with rest and relaxation.

Majority of the Alzheimer's patients do live at home with their loved ones and family in the U.S. It is simply untrue that most Americans abandon their impaired, sick elderly parents to die at the long-term facilities or nursing homes. Many social studies have shown that many spouses and adult children are taking care of their aging and memory-impaired spouses and parents or grandparents in the same household under one roof; those who do not live together are closely involved in the care of their family who have Alzheimer's disease. Of course, you can find a few who do not wish to be the caregivers due to various reasons, most families are usually trying and doing their best at great personal sacrifice to provide suitable care for their family members with Alzheimer's.

Undoubtedly, watching someone close to you decline mentally and physically in a slow motion can be a grueling struggle and a painful experience. Inherently, this involves also in changes in roles and added responsibilities for everyone in the family in relation to the impaired member, who can be the spouse, grandparent, parent, or older sister and older brother. A change in the role generally means new and additional responsibility. It is very important for every caregiver to understand that the impaired individual acts as he or she does because he or she is sick and cannot help themselves. Sometimes, that person you are helping does not look sick even though parts of the brain have been damaged.

By 'role', it means a person's place in the family. Roles are usually and traditionally established over many years, and defined by certain responsibilities or tasks. With the loved one suffering from Alzheimer's disease, a dementing illness, sometimes problems seem insurmountable because they involve and require both changes in roles and the need for you to learn new tasks. Having to learn new skills and assume new responsibilities when you are overwhelmed and frustrated can be difficult.

There are many real-life examples: a spouse who has never managed the check-book may feel that he or she does not have the ability to manage money. Or an impaired husband can no longer do the carving of a turkey at the Thanksgiving dinner, the wife or adult children have to learn the skill of carving the turkey. Or the well husband has to do the laundry, learning not to mix colored items with white ones. Or a wife who has been driven with and by the husband most of her life, now she has to do all the driving since her husband gave up his job due to Alzheimer's disease.

The adult children and the father have to learn to make suppers and do the grocery shopping because the children's mother is now unable to cook and take care of many household chores due to her impaired memory and dementia. The ill and dementing wife may rely on her husband and children to take a bath and change the clothes totally as the disease progresses. You must try to retain her dignity at the same time that you and other family members provided her with the needed care.

When a man realizes that he is not the head of the family, his abilities are waning and becoming more dependent, he may be discouraged, angry and depressed. The family and caregivers should help him maintain his role and position as an important member of the family even when he cannot do the tasks he once did. You should continue to consult him, involve him in conversations, and listen to him attentively, even if what he says may seem confounded. Let him know by these actions and interactions that he is still respected.

Occasionally, your beloved wife with Alzheimer's disease will insist that you are not her husband; It must be very heart-breaking for the caregiver-husband in such a difficult and sad situation. All you can do is to reassure your impaired spouse, "I am your husband", but avoid arguing. You also need to reassure yourself that it is not a rejection of you. It is just an inexplicable confusion of your spouse's brain.

Sometimes, a caregiver may feel that the impaired person is "seeing the dead". Perhaps, the memory of a dear dead person is stronger than the memory of the death. This is a general feeling of loss by the impaired person with Alzheimer's, and your contradicting and arguing with that person with a dementing illness can make matter worse, or may even lead to a catastrophic reaction. Instead, ask the impaired individual about the deceased, or look through a photo album, or re-tell some old family stories. This is not 'spooky' and the issue is not worth the argument.

There is a phenomenon called dementia-related psychosis, and this symptom is not uncommon in people suffering from Alzheimer's disease, Lewy body dementia, vascular dementia and dementia related to Parkinson's disease. The psychosis symptoms and behaviors include hallucination, delusional thinking, agitation and aggressive acting-out. They are usually seen during the advanced or final stages of the disease process.

The impaired person may have visual, auditory, or olfactory hallucinations --- seeing, hearing or smelling things that are not there. These can be disruptive sometimes, requiring treatment; but if the impaired person sees a tiger in the living room and it does not bother him or her, that hallucination may need to be treated. For the caregivers, maintaining a calm, serene demeanor is always helpful when the impaired person is experiencing dementia-related psychosis. Many experts agree that medication should not be the first step; it is imperative to find out what might be going on to cause the psychosis and make sure that the 'sick' individual is engaged.

In the final stages of the dementing illness, most, if not all of the patients have to be institutionalized. Among the different deteriorating bodily functions, their vision can be severely impaired despite fitting eye-glasses because the patients are just unable to process the images received any more. They are becoming harder and harder to reach by the devoted, loving caregivers. Some family-caregivers might try to bring them home once in a while for an overnight visit and bonding, but the family often found the experience of getting together very heart-sick and the pain and anguish unbearable.

A personal note from the author:

My wife sustained a major stroke in the year 2018; she has had long history of hypertension, diabetes, hyperlipidemia, and mildly overweight. Her post-CVA MRI scans revealed, among other pertinent findings, depositions of amyloids. With her multiple contributing risk factors and clinical manifestations after the stroke, I firmly believe that she is suffering from Alzheimer's disease in its early stages in the midst of her other co-morbidities.

She worked in my two medical offices part-time to handle the general managerial and administrative matters until my medical license was suspended and I was indicted by Federal DEA for prescribing controlled substances (opioid analgesics), "illegitimately", meaning for patients who did not have legitimate diagnoses or pain requiring opioid analgesics, despite the medical records demonstrating multiple, documented painful conditions and diagnoses.

Anyway, as a caregiver for a mentally-impaired person, you cannot expect logics or the so-called 'common senses'. I have to take over any cooking involving the gas-stove or range at home because of the incident of intense smoke and nearly fire due to her forgetting something she put on the stove. She is told that she can use the microwave for heating certain foods and drinks; even then, the items in the microwave can get too hot, too dry and burnt sometimes. With her urinary and occasional fecal incontinence, with the precise etiology unknown, sometimes, she will walk on the urine on the floor when the diapers worn are totally soaked. That is why, I try to remind her of the bathroom needs every 2 to 3 hours. Doing laundry at home has become routine for me after work when our part-time house-keeper is gone for the day. Needless to say, I have been her personal driver as needed. My 62-year- old wife used to remember the telephone numbers of all of her family and good friends, and reluctant to take advantage of caller ID/speed dial. Of course, now, she has to rely on the contacts for speed dial because remembering their numbers seem to be more difficult especially when she dials more and more wrong numbers.

Our modern technology is wonderful, and many of us are satisfied with and grateful for it because it does save time and provides much information quickly. But, getting away from memorizing the telephone numbers of friends and family members and solely dependent on speed dials may not be good for brain health. Instead of evolving, you may be devolving from the perspective of memory. I do have most, if not all of the telephone numbers used regularly on speed dial, but I always say the numbers quietly before the calls, and so far, so good. There are just too many nuances and things to describe and talk about when you are a caregiver for someone with Alzheimer's disease.

POST-SURGICAL DELIRIUM AND ALZHEIMER'S

Post-surgical delirium is a common, if not the most common, post-operative complication in older adults. By definition, delirium is a serious disruption in mental abilities that results in unclear or confused thinking, reduced awareness of the surroundings, restlessness and anxiety, delusions, incoherence, and sometimes hallucination. Its onset can be a few hours or a few days after surgery.

Three types of delirium have been identified:

- Hyperactive delirium with agitation, restlessness, irritability, combativeness and sometimes hallucination.

- Hypoactive delirium with lethargy, sluggishness, drowsiness and reduced motor activity.

- Mixed delirium with both hyper- and hypo-active states. The affected person may switch back and forth from hyperactive to hypoactive states.

There are a few contributing factors, such as chronic illness, infection, and sensory deprivations (blindness or deafness). Other causative factors, though not post-surgical, include alcohol or drug intoxication or withdrawal.

According to the most recent statistics, about 4 to 5 adults in the U.S. hospitals become delirious every minute after surgeries under general anesthesia. These high figures are astounding, adding up to 2.5 to 2.6 million cases annually of post-surgical delirium. Most medical professionals regard post-surgical delirium as a 'normal' but temporary state with little or without any long-term impact because the symptoms generally only last a short time, maybe three to four days post-operatively.

However, some older patients could not even remember their birthdays or what country they were in beyond the three-four days after surgery. Researchers noticed that many, with follow-up studies, showed continued decline of their cognitive ability with a diagnosis of Alzheimer's disease one year after the incident of post-surgical delirium.

We must admit that post-surgical delirium is probably more prevalent than people realize, and must not minimize its profound negative impact on mental health. Unfortunately, its causes are not clear at this time; anesthesia during surgery may play a role according to some researchers. Patients become unconscious under general anesthesia. In post-anesthetic unconscious state, the neurons of different senses do not stop firing and their activities can be demonstrated in brain-wave studies. In reality and actuality, patients' connectivity are subdued or suppressed during sedation by general anesthesia. During post-operative recovery, most patients are able to resume normal brain activities, but in some post-op patients, I believe that the connectivity in the brain are unfortunately compromised.

Beyond the possible adverse effects of general anesthesia, anxiety in general, along with post-operative medications such as opioid analgesics and sedatives may be involved. Any unsuspected, pre-existing neurodegenerative disorders can be a major risk for the development of post-surgical delirium. Nevertheless, the current statistics for the high number of cases are just mind-boggling and hard to accept passively. We must all strive to reduce and avoid if possible the incidents of post-surgical delirium, and not to consider and accept them as temporary conditions after surgeries, because these cases can have far-reaching, devastating effects on the patients and their families and our society as whole.

Immediate attention should be focused on patients' post-operative nutritional support, the avoidance of mind-altering medications, appropriate brain stimulations such as eye-glasses and hearing aids, and their surroundings which promote restful sleep.

Before surgery, it is prudent and important that patient and family should convene including the attending physicians and designated surgeon to discuss the risks and types of anesthesia for the surgical procedure, especially an elective operation. Anesthesiologists or anesthetists should be present at the meeting to educate and answer questions. More and more medical institutions, including medical schools and hospitals have accepted and used acupunctural anesthesia for certain surgical procedures.

It is my sincere advice that any adult, who is contemplating and considering surgery, major or minor, that requires general anesthesia, should be proactive and concerned, together with your family and loved ones to become educated medical consumers. After all, it is your life and your brain, and life without a normal, functioning brain is no life at all!

For older adults who are going to have elective surgeries requiring general anesthesia, a pre-surgical screening along with a mini-mental status examination should be performed by qualified medical professionals or psychologists to have a baseline prior to the surgery. Furthermore, you should start or continue your healthy lifestyle with regular exercise, proper nutrition and adequate sleep to prepare yourself for the surgery and to minimize the risk of post-surgical delirium.

Any surgical procedure carries some risk and nobody can guarantee it risk-free; however, everyone should be aware of the possibility of post-surgical delirium and its possible impact on increasing the risk for the development of Alzheimer's disease. Therefore, as a preventive protocol, a careful and in-depth pre-surgical assessment is crucial with collaboration of the medical team consisting of attending physician, designated surgeon, anesthesiologist or anesthetist and qualified psychologist.

ALZHEIMER'S DISEASE AND NUTRITION

"Let food be your only medicine!" by Hippocrates (460-377 BCE).

For many years, the main-stream medicine had ignored and/or down-played the important role diet could play in both health and diseases. More recently, with increasing plethora of evidence for the positive and beneficial impacts of certain nutrients on many illnesses, the medical establishments have begun to emphasize the importance and need to eat healthy foods to keep diseases at bay.

With aging, our ability to absorb nutrients in the gastrointestinal tract decreases. The intestinal tract has millions of nerves, more than the spinal cord; and the digestive system produces just as many neurotransmitters as the brain. It is no wonder that some people are referring to the intestinal tract as the body's second brain. Furthermore, it is undeniable and clear that certain nutrients play essential roles in neural development and functions.

To get the most out of the nutritious diets, especially the older population, we must ensure that the intestinal tract is competent with the full team of beneficial bacteria (microbiome) performing optimally. The geriatric population, those with the diagnosis of Alzheimer's disease, or the suspicion thereof, have special needs for particular nutrients. Let us review briefly the digestive process, starting with chewing the food in the mouth.

It is important for older individuals to have functional and healthy dentition to enjoy all healthy foods. After swallowing, the food is pushed down to the stomach through the esophagus. Then, the muscles lining the digestive tract continually move the partially digested foods into and through the intestines via peristalsis. The small intestine, which is about 16 to 20 feet long, is responsible for the absorption of most of the nutrients, The villi and microvilli of the intestinal lining, essentially innumerable, absorb the nutrients from the foods and make them available to the bloodstream. Waste products that cannot be used, such as undigested food, are pushed down into the colon and finally expelled from the rectum.

At least 65 to 70% of our immune system is located in and around the digestive systems, and our health is dependent upon the trillions of bacteria in the guts, called microbiome. The microbial flora in our intestines perform many beneficial functions for the body: they produce vitamins which include biotin, thiamine, riboflavin, niacin, pantothenic acid, pyridoxin, cobalamin. folic acid and vitamin K. The microbial flora also help improve the absorption of many nutrients such as calcium, copper, iron, magnesium, manganese and some vitamins. So, one important way to boost and enhance the immune system is to protect and improve the integrity of the microbiome of the guts, and this can be achieved by adding live probiotics.

"You are what you eat" is a proverbial adage with true and profound significance. Food is an important part of good health, not just for survival; and it is one that you have control over and can do something about. Nutrients from food, especially in its natural, wholesome forms, are the best fuels that power the body and mind, maintaining good physical and mental health and vitality.

Experts recommend eating mostly of the foods that help keep the body in an alkaline state, because an acidic condition or milieu tends to make the body more susceptible and prone to illnesses. Studies have shown that a 75 to 80% plant-based diet of fruits and vegetables helps shift the body's chemistry toward a predominantly alkaline state. As an added benefit, this plant-based diet facilitates elimination; constipation is a common complaint among the elderly people, and a balance between assimilation and elimination is vitally important for the body to maintain homeostasis and optimal health.

As a reminder, do not prepare and cook your food in any aluminum utensils due to a possible link between aluminum poisoning and Alzheimer's disease and similar form of dementia. Autopsies performed on Alzheimer's patients revealed higher levels of aluminum in many of their brain tissues. Instead of aluminum cook-wares, switch to using glass, ceramic or stainless steel for your cooking.

Specifically, there is no such a thing as an Alzheimer's diet, but eating a Mediterranean diet seems to be a universally accepted, positive strategy. The Mediterranean diet is not a fad; it is a lifestyle choice, involving most of the foods available in a sustainable way. The famous diet is plant-heavy with vegetables, fruits, wholegrains, fish and pulses. Olive oil, with healthy fat, is used almost exclusively, while lemons are common staples in the kitchen. Red wine in not excluded in moderation. For the history buff, Mediterranean diet is believed to have started in Crete, Greece, a historically rich island.

Researchers at Rush Alzheimer's Disease Center in Chicago created the MIND diet, short for Mediterranean-Dash Intervention for Neurodegenerative Disease (or Delay) with ten beneficial foods as follows:

- Berries, especially blueberries
- Beans
- Fatty fish (including crustaceans)
- Olive oil
- Poultry (non-fried)
- Nuts
- Vegetables (dark green and leafy)
- Hard-boiled eggs, 4 to 5 times a week
- Whole grains
- Red wine (resveratrol)

Researchers from Chicago Rush University Medical Center found that adding in foods like pizza, sweets and pastries with added sugar, processed meats, fried things like French Fries, and sodas reversed the cognitive benefits from the Mediterranean diet. Their studies examined more than 5,000 seniors over three years and found that those who stuck to the Mediterranean diet had brains that were nearly six years younger than their peers who gave in to junk food cravings.

According to the findings from recent studies, researchers have found a link between eating a Mediterranean-style diet and delayed onset of Parkinson's disease. The delayed onset can be as much as 17 years of Parkinson's disease, a progressive neurodegenerative disease. In other words, the researchers support that adherence to the Mediterranean or MIND diet can reduce the incidence and delay the progression of neurodegenerative diseases such as Alzheimer's and Parkinson's.

It is not surprising from the plethora of supportive and encouraging evidence that Mediterranean diet is now considered to be an important modifiable factor in Alzheimer's disease. In a 2013 study of 550 people aged between 55 and 80 by researchers in Spain, the participants were randomly assigned either a low-fat diet plan or a Mediterranean diet. They followed their assigned diets for 6.5 years; the follow-up results showed that those who ate a Mediterranean diet scored the highest on cognitive tests.

A 5-year-long study of 960 adults aged 81 and older who were dementia-free at the start of the study was published in the journal of the Alzheimer's Association; the researchers remarkably found that those who followed the MIND diet to the letter dramatically reduced their risk of Alzheimer's disease by as much as 53%. For those who did not adhere to the MIND diet whole-heartedly on a daily basis still reduced their risk of the disease by 35%.

Several recent studies by other researchers revealed that the brains of healthy, middle-aged individuals who faithfully followed the Mediterranean or MIND diet had less atrophy on the MRI brain scans and less accumulation of the beta-amyloid protein than people who did not follow the specific diet regimen. Most experts and researchers seem to agree that the Mediterranean diet is able to positively influence inflammation and oxidative stress in the brain, lowering their levels and reducing the formation of plaques and tangles that cause damages in the neurons of people with Alzheimer's disease.

According to a new study published by the University of Edinburgh, the Mediterranean diet is also linked to better thinking skills later in life, i.e. it can keep you mentally sharp. The researchers tested over 500 people all at the age of 79, and without dementia. The participants completed numerous tests to evaluate their problem solving, thinking speed, memory and word knowledge along with MRI scans. The results of this study showed that people who adhered closer to a Mediterranean diet had higher scores for cognitive functions. In particular, the individual diet components that stood out to the researchers were higher consumption of leafy green vegetables and lower consumption of red meat.

Researchers at the German Center for Neurodegenerative Diseases in Bonn studied the brain scans of more than 500 older adults who ate a Mediterranean diet and found that they were less likely to show brain shrinkage and high levels of abnormal proteins, amyloids. Adhering to a Mediterranean diet could help slow down Alzheimer's disease and prevent cognitive decline, as they reported these findings in the medical journal 'Neurology'.

When the researchers analyzed the combined results of the brain scans, cognitive tests and diet scores along with demographic factors such as sex, age and education, they further found that each point lower on the dietary score actually corresponded to almost one year of brain aging. Moreover, those who had lower dietary scores, meaning not adhering to the Mediterranean diet faithfully, were more likely to have lower scores on memory tests and to have higher levels of amyloid and tau.

The Mediterranean diet must act on specific mechanisms related to the neuropathology of Alzheimer's disease by modulating neuro-inflammation and reducing the oxidative stress, and sustaining brain health through beneficial systemic effects, fostering and enhancing cardiovascular and brain health.

I feel it necessary to point out some impressive studies about the neuro-protective properties of blueberries. The studies were done by researchers at the University of Cincinnati, the U.S. Department of Agriculture, and the Canadian Department of Agriculture in 2010, on participants in their 70s with symptoms of memory loss. One group was given blueberry juice everyday for two months, while the other half of subjects were given look-alike substitute. When testing was concluded, the participants with the blueberries had improved their performance considerably on the memory tests, whereas the other group showed no changes.

In general, all the berries are good for the brain; they include blackberries, strawberries, raspberries, and blueberries in particular. Berries are one of the best sources of antioxidants with high concentrations of antioxidant and anti-inflammatory phytochemicals. These bioactive phytochemicals are powerful reducers of oxidative and inflammatory stresses, able to prevent or delay aging, especially the brain, protecting you against age-related cognitive decline.

The "Free Radical" is one of the widely accepted theories on aging. Free radicals can adversely affect or damage DNA, causing genetic mutations. Most of the free radicals of biological significance are simply reactive forms of molecular oxygen; it is paradoxical, ironic and perplexing that oxygen is not only necessary for life, but it is also the primary cause of aging and eventual death.

The human body generates free radicals continuously inside every cell with the biochemical reactions. Normally, most of these free radicals are neutralized by antioxidants defenses; when these defenses are compromised, the build-up of free radicals can cause damage to tissues, cells and their vital cellular components such as DNA and proteins. This gradual physiological deterioration over time is referred to as 'aging', according to one theory. One of the harmful free radical influences is misfolding of proteins, resulting in biological abnormalities such as formation of beta-amyloid plaques and Tau neuro-fibrillary tangles.

When Hippocrates, thousands of years ago, said, "Let food be your only medicine! ", his observation and wise suggestion should be taken seriously. With the complexity, pace and dense populations of our modern cities, and the man-made pollution of the environments, a well-balanced, nutritious diet is certainly important to help fight many ailments and diseases, but it is only a part of the wellness equation.

When a person sustains a stroke, heart attack or head trauma hard enough to injure the brain cells, this undoubtedly interrupts the flow of oxygenated blood to the brain and the neurons begin to die within minutes. Generally speaking, health care providers always ensure an adequate oxygen supply for patients, but often neglect the importance and need of timely, adequate nutrition, either intravenous or through a G-tube. After an injury, major one in particular, the body essentially enters a hyper-metabolic state, requiring more calories than normal to provide the energy and nutrients to rebuild damaged tissues, especially the brain. In fact, feeding patients with brain injuries is so important that neurologists have actually put some remarkable numbers to it: The 5,7,2,4,100,200 solution:

Patients with brain injury who are not fed nutritiously within 5 days after head trauma are two times more likely to die than are patients who get fed. Post-trauma patients, if not fed within 7 days are four times more likely to die than are patients who get fed. The best menu is to provide 100% of the normal daily calories for that patient; up to 200% is even better. Starting to feed patients with brain injuries aggressively at the earliest outset possible is now recognized as one of the most important factors improving outcome. In fact, we have been able to reduce mortality, minimize damage and improve outcome in patients with head trauma over the past two decades by maintaining their blood pressures and supplying the body and the brain early on with oxygen and nutrients.

The Alzheimer's patients are generally under-nourished with inadequate nutrients and fluid (water). Their brains, essentially, are in chronic injured state, requiring sufficient nutrition for optimal tissue repair and outcome.

Researchers in England, neutral and non-partisan, examined the mortality of 11,000 people recruited through health-food stores and vegetarian societies in a 17-year study, and found that their mortality was half that of the general population. The researchers who carried out the studies at the Radcliffe Infirmary in Oxford published the findings in the British Medical Journal. Clearly, the benefits of fruits and vegetables are indisputable.

According to the CDC, less than 10% of Americans (adults and children) eat the recommended amount of vegetables, and this is a pretty sad statistic. There are so many health reasons why you should be eating vegetables, though most of you probably already know, but they are worth repeating. People may wonder how many vegetables they need to eat per day, actually, it is not as much as you would think. According to the USDA Dietary Guidelines, for an average adult, women or men, we need three to four cups of vegetables each day. It is easy to break down your vegetable intake by meal; simply add a serving to every meal and you will reach your daily recommendation in no time. Fresh vegetables are not the only way you can get and accomplish your daily servings; canned and frozen veggies are also nutritious alternatives as long as there are no added sugars.

Manufacturing and marketing of vitamin and mineral supplements is a multibillion dollar industry, nowadays. I am not a supporter of indiscriminate and excessive use of supplemental vitamins and minerals, because some of them such as the fat-soluble ones, vitamin A, D, E, and K which can cause cumulative toxicities with serious, harmful effects to the human body. Even if others that are water-soluble, non-judicious, excessive and superfluous consumption is not wise and unnecessary for people who have a balanced diet with 75 to 80% of fruits and vegetables. In fact, some of these water-soluble ones can also cause some health issues.

If one has a special medical need for certain vitamin, such as vitamin B12 for pernicious anemia, or people with neurodegenerative diseases like Alzheimer's who can benefit from neuroprotective nutrients, a few of these are presented in the following texts with documented, impartial studies despite some skeptic minds. Again, sensible, judicious and educated use of supplemental vitamins and minerals is advised in cooperation with your physician and/or professional dietician and nutritionist.

It is difficult to persuade the general population, especially the children to faithfully follow a diet which is 75 to 80% of fruits and vegetables. The ubiquitous and tempting commercial advertisements of fast and convenient, and somewhat delicious-looking foods are, no doubt, making it harder for many people.

There are three amino acids, leucine, isoleucine and valine, which are important for memory and cognition. They share a distinct chemical structure - a long central chain with smaller side chains branching out – they are called branched chain amino acids (BCAA). The body uses the BCAAs to build neurotransmitters, and injured brain often suffer reduced levels of leucine, isoleucine and valine. Neuroscientists added BCAAs to the drinking water of brain-injured mice and observed improvements in both memory and cognition. Follow-up studies also showed that the three amino acids seemed to help 'wakefulness', the ability to stay awake and alert, after some brain trauma applied to the mice. BCAAs should be beneficial for humans, especially people with Alzheimer's and TBI, who have nothing to lose.

Vitamin C:

It is such a famous nutrient with believers and skeptics for its health benefits. Vitamin C (ascorbic acid) is a water-soluble antioxidant, which helps the body get rid of undesirable and harmful chemicals, the free radicals, that damage the cells and DNA. Humans have lost the ability of making vitamin C, which is an essential micronutrient, and we must get it from the diets. We have the genes that are necessary for the synthesis of vitamin C, but one of them is mutated; this mutated or broken gene known as GULO, codes for an enzyme that is necessary for a key step in vitamin C synthesis.

Vitamin C is an integral part of many structures of our body, and the body cannot make collagen without vitamin C working as a co-factor, and it would fall apart without the protein collagen. In the body, collagen fibers are the most important, structural and shock-absorbing component of the connective tissues. Collagen fibers twist around each other to form the scaffolding for the bones, cartilages, skin and muscles (including the muscles of the heart). Collagen is also the supportive component of ligaments, tendons and blood vessels. Collagen keeps your skin from getting wrinkles; you need collagen to grow new skin and form scar tissue when you get a cut.

In fact, vitamin C is necessary to make key hormones that carry signals from your brain all over the body; these hormones include but not limited to serotonin, dopamine, epinephrine and nor-epinephrine. Vitamin C comes from fruits and vegetables, including oranges and bell peppers. Most people who eat a variety of fruits and vegetables daily should have enough of this vitamin from their foods with a healthy lifestyle. Smokers are found to have lower levels of vitamin C than non-smokers because of the considerable amounts of free radicals generated by cigarette smoking. Vitamin C is vulnerable to heat and destroyed by oxygen, and losses of vitamin can be expected when a food is stored, cut, heated or processed, resulting in some reduced levels in the body.

The safe range of vitamin C intake seems to be broad and somewhat controversial, as opposed to the daily recommended guideline by the U.S. Government. The optimal physiological amount of vitamin C varies among different individuals, depending on one's lifestyle and health conditions. In general, doses approaching 8 to 10 grams a day can be expected to be unsafe, causing problems such as kidney stones, and hemochromatosis (Vitamin C promotes the absorption of iron from the intestines and its excessive supplement may be dangerous for people already with an overload of iron in the body). At massive doses, vitamin C may unwittingly counteract the effect of anti-clotting medications.

Tom Kirkwood, an eminent researcher on aging at the University of Newcastle gave a vivid depiction of the action of vitamin C in 2001:

"When a molecule of vitamin C encounters a free radical, it becomes oxidized and thereby renders the free radical innocuous. The oxidized vitamin C molecule then gets restored to its non-oxidized state by an enzyme called vitamin C reductase." As we know, some vitamin C is degraded irretrievably and must be replaced, even though some is recycled back to its active form for re-use.

Researchers at Cambridge in 2001 reported in the Lancet that the risk of death from any cause was higher in people with low plasma levels of vitamin C, and conversely, that people with high plasma levels of vitamin C were less likely to die within the period studied. The studies seem to imply that vitamin C lengthens life span. However, the researchers were careful to point out that there was no association between vitamin C supplementation and mortality, and the linkage is generally with dietary intake from fresh, canned or frozen sources.

Linus Pauling, a 2-time Nobel laureate and the distinguished Scottish oncologist, Evan Cameron, reported that mega-doses of vitamin C, given intravenously could quadruple the survival time of patients with advanced cancer, even bringing about complete remission in some cases.

Scurvy is no longer familiar sight, but once a scourge, devastating the lives of sailors, who were deprived of fresh foods including vegetables on their long voyages. These afflicted individuals suffered weakened limbs which became swollen and discolored while their gums bled profusely. Other symptoms included easy bruising, anemia, fatigue, heart failure and eventually death.

In the absence of vitamin C, collagen fibers do not form properly. As a result, blood vessels become fragile and wounds heal slowly, if at all. The bleeding gum, and spontaneous easy bruising can occur anywhere in the body. Vitamin C also acts on the inorganic iron in food in the intestinal tract, converting iron from the insoluble form found in food (Fe^{3+}) to the soluble, usable form (Fe^{2+}) which can then be absorbed into the bloodstream. Without adequate supply of vitamin C, one cannot absorb enough iron to stock the red blood cells with hemoglobin, leading to anemia. That is why anemia is a treatable cause of impaired memory.

The U.S. recommended daily allowance (RDA) for an average normal adult is about 100mg; this value can vary when special needs of one's body is considered.

There is no question that un-neutralized accumulation of superfluous free radicals produced in the body are associated with aging and chronic degenerative diseases, and their deleterious attacks on the cells, cellular constituents like DNA, and connective tissues are well-documented. The damages caused by free radicals to cell membranes, proteins and DNA can be measured with growing refinement over the past decade.

Many antioxidants require "partner" antioxidants allowing them to work more efficiently, e.g. vitamin C and E, selenium and co-enzyme Q10.

Vitamin E:

Many experts agree that the fat-soluble vitamin E is a strong defender of the cell membrane because it plays an essential role in protecting lipids, the major component of cell membranes, from oxidation. Vitamin E donates electrons directly to the free radicals, rendering them innocuous and harmless.

When vitamin E reacts and neutralize a free radical, it becomes a weakly reactive free radical product, called alpha-tocopheryl. This is then re-converted into stable vitamin E again by accepting electrons from vitamin C. The more the vitamin C available, the quicker the regeneration of vitamin E for antioxidant activities. Free radicals, if left unchecked, cause heightened inflammation.

White blood cells that fight diseases depend on vitamin E to bolster our defense. The chemically reactive free radicals, when unchecked, can initiate a rapid destructive chain reaction, resulting in:

- Cell membrane lipid damage
- Cellular protein damage
- DNA damage
- Oxidation of LDL-cholesterol
- Inflammation

Antioxidants, such as vitamin E, can stop and modify this destructive chain reaction by changing the nature of the free radicals. Vitamin E from foods is generally safe to consume; toxicity usually comes from supplements. To err on the safe side, people who use vitamin E supplements should keep their dosages low. When in doubt, it is prudent and important to consult with your physician and/or nutritionist to avoid any potential adverse side effects.

Vitamin E supplements, as many studies have shown, can augment the effects of anti-coagulant medications prescribed to oppose unwanted clotting of blood for patients who need blood thinners under the supervision of the prescribing doctors. At high doses, vitamin E can inhibit the aggregation of platelets and block the clotting activities of vitamin K. So, you must exercise extreme care and caution when considering vitamin E supplementation if you are on any types of anti-coagulation therapy including aspirin, not to risk any uncontrollable hemorrhage. One study has revealed that an increase in brain hemorrhage, a form of stroke, is noted among some smokers taking daily vitamin E, even at 50mg per day. The Office of

Supplements suggests that the maximum safe daily intake for most adults is 1,000mg of vitamin E per day.

One study that was published in the New England Journal of Medicine involved some selected subjects and treated them with higher doses of vitamin E in relation to its anti-inflammatory properties to slow the progression of Alzheimer's disease. The findings in this particular study seemed to have revealed some promise. Researchers have shown that vitamin E and CoQ10 work synergistically; each is required for re-generation of the other. Clinically, their combination works better than either alone. In addition to CoQ10, vitamin E also requires adequate selenium for optimal antioxidant effects. Selenium is a component of the antioxidant enzyme, glutathione peroxidase, which works with vitamin E to enhance their beneficial effects, preventing free radicals from damaging the cell membranes.

Some other studies have shown that antioxidants may shield the ApoE4 protein from oxidative stress, and vitamin E stands out in the studies, and is proven to delay or postpone the onset of Alzheimer's disease, or slow its progression. There are quite a few good sources of vitamin E, and these include sunflower seeds, almonds, avocados, kiwi, peanuts, dark leafy greens such as spinach, and some oils. In terms of vitamin E from fruits, avocados is at the top, a super food and a rich source of vitamin E in addition to other nutrients such as vitamin C, folic acid and many B vitamins.

Avocado also provides lutein, a carotenoid pigment which is important for vision, and beta-carotene, another carotenoid that the body converts to a form of vitamin A. Vision is one of the important senses, probably the most important one for brain stimulation. People who eat foods rich in lutein and zeaxanthin are less likely to develop age-related macular degeneration, the leading cause of blindness in older adults. Avocado is also a good source of dietary fiber, and the heart- and brain-healthy omega-3 fatty acids. Indeed, avocado should be a super-choice of food to help fight against Alzheimer's disease.

According to Dr. Dale Bredesen, a renowned researcher for Alzheimer's disease, "Alzheimer's disease is not a mysterious, untreatable brain disease; it is a reversible, metabolic systemic illness with a relatively large window for treatment."

It is worth repeating that chronic hyperinsulinemia is a risk factor for Alzheimer's disease. Carbohydrates and sugar seem to continue to represent the foundation of the modern American diet, not anywhere near the healthy, highly-recommended 75 to 80% of fruits and vegetables. Most people do not realize that over time, the high carbohydrate diet will have devastating effects on our general health, including the brain.

When there is too much in the blood, the hemoglobin, which is a protein carrying oxygen in the blood, become sticky with the sugar --- a glycated hemoglobin. This dysfunctional hemoglobin then result in poor delivery of oxygen and nutrients to different tissues, including the brain. Hemoglobin is not the only protein molecules in the body that can be glycated; sometimes. The glycated molecules bond with each other, forming larger groups called Advanced Glycation End products (AGEs).

The proteins in the neurons are susceptible to glycation damage when exposed to chronic hyper-glycemia, compromising transmission of nerve impulses and increasing the risk of Alzheimer's disease.

Oxidative stress occurs when there is an imbalance in the equilibrium between ROS production and the antioxidant defense system. An increase in oxidative stress from excessive free radicals accelerates aging and vulnerability of the brain. Oxidative stress inherently may also induce the expression of pro-inflammatory cytokines, thus raising the levels of inflammation. The phenomenon of inflammation in Alzheimer's disease is well established.

Many studies have suggested that inflammatory events in the CNS may have an important role in exaggerating or increasing neuronal deficits in aging. Activated glial cells of the brain are associated with inflammation, and their activation is considered the hallmark of inflammation in the brain. The activated microglia produce pro-inflammatory cytokines such as interleukin-1 (IL-1), interleukin-6 IL-6), and tumor necrosis factor-alpha (TNF-alpha), forming a feedback loop to perpetuate and amplify the inflammatory signaling cascade.

Researchers in neuroscience seem to have suggested that one method to forestall or perhaps even reverse the declines in aging and Alzheimer's disease is to increase the endogenous antioxidant and anti-inflammatory protection, thus decreasing and minimizing the vulnerability of the brain. There is an inverse relationship between the levels of antioxidant/anti-inflammatory and the vulnerability factor of the Central Nervous System. The harmful effects of oxidative stress with damage to DNA, protein oxidation, membrane lipid peroxidation, and abnormal sequestration of metals may be independent of beta-amyloid deposition.

Nevertheless, there is undoubtedly an increased vulnerability to oxidative stress and inflammatory insults in senescence, more so in individuals with Alzheimer's disease. Both free radicals and oxidative stress play a crucial role in the pathophysiology of neurodegenerative diseases such as Alzheimer's and Parkinson's diseases with an increase in the production of inflammatory mediators. Moreover, the important roles played by the glial cells of the brain are becoming more remarkable and clearer, supporting the survival of the neurons.

Again, the importance of a plant-based diet for human health is indisputable. In the case of fruits and vegetables, their composition is not limited to their macronutrients (carbohydrates, proteins, and fats) and micronutrients (vitamins and minerals). They contain another class of molecules found in significant amounts: phytochemical compounds.

Polyphenols are in the largest class of phytochemical compounds, and the brightly colored fruits and vegetables are major sources of polyphenols. The phytochemical compounds produced by plants have anti-bacterial, anti-fungal and insecticidal functions that minimize any harm caused by attackers and allow the plants to survive in hostile conditions. In general, phytochemicals are not involved in their primary metabolism; they have other functions such as enhancing the plants' survivability. They can function positively, modulating the environment of the cells including neurons to keep them in a latent, harmless state.

Many recent studies have shown that many phytochemical compounds play a front-line role in the body's defense system against chronic diseases including cancers and neurodegenerative disorders. Polyphenols have a chemical structure that is ideal for absorbing or neutralizing free radicals, and some of them are actually more powerful than vitamin C.

Researchers have recently found that polyphenols have shown considerable efficacy in reducing the deleterious effects of neuronal aging and in maintaining the health of neurons. Many polyphenols have been identified to date, and here are just a few of the common, important ones:

- Curcumin in turmeric
- Resveratrol in grapes
- Catechins in green tea
- Genistein in soybeans
- Ellagic acid in strawberries and raspberries
- Delphinidin in blueberries

Generally speaking, for older adults, especially for individuals with Alzheimer's disease, in my opinion, the macronutrient ratios should be:

- Healthy fats: 50 to 55%
- Quality proteins: 25 to 30%
- Carbohydrates: 20 to 25%

Most people, if not everyone, essentially agree that a plant-based diet consisting of 75 to 80% vegetables and fruits is beneficial for our general health and well-being. Some individuals with the diagnosis of Alzheimer's disease and their caregivers and families wonder if there are certain foods that may be more specifically nutritious and supportive from the perspectives of Alzheimer's disease. I am going to list some foods that can be helpful and should be incorporated into the diet for the Alzheimer's patients while maintaining a balanced plant-based daily menu. These foods are recognized as beneficial with support from the scientific data; but, not an attestation to the cause-and-effect relationships.

- Blueberries (Berries)
- Spinach and broccoli (and other dark-green, leafy vegetables)
- Lamb
- SMASH (Sardines, Mackerel, Anchovies, Salmon and Herrings)
- Dark chocolate in moderation
- Green or white tea
- Eggs
- Beets
- Walnuts
- Black beans
- Tomatoes
- Oranges and apples (of low glycemic index)
- Turmeric
- Poultry (quality protein instead of red meat)
- Whole grains
- Olive oil
- Avocado
- Grapes and pomegranates

A special note: A prudent, plant-based diet is one of the best defenses against the development of Alzheimer's disease. One of the foods is the packaged buttered popcorn, which contains a common additive for its buttery flavor called Diacetyl. Diacetyl is naturally produced by fermentation processes, but is also frequently synthesized by chemical manufacturers for its use as a food additive. Recent studies by researchers at the University of Minnesota through the Chemical Research in Toxicology Journal have linked Diacetyl to the development of beta amyloids in the brain, and by association, the development of Alzheimer's disease. Thus, avoiding the regular consumption of foods that contain Diacetyl will not guarantee that you will not develop Alzheimer's disease, but it can help decrease the buildup of beta amyloids associated with it.

A note regarding the red wine in the Mediterranean diet if you are a wine drinker: needless to say, moderation is recommended with one glass for the women and up to two glasses for the men daily. The phenolic compounds in the red wine possess antioxidant and anti-inflammatory properties, and have been shown to reduce oxidative stress. In a 2019 study published in "Gastroenterology", it revealed that those who drank red wine had a more diverse and healthier gut microbiota, compared to subjects non-drinkers of red wine. The effect was not observed among those who drank white wine, beer or spirits. Many neuroscientists and researchers have found links between unfriendly gut bacteria and degenerative brain disorders such as Alzheimer's disease, Parkinson's disease and amyotrophic Lateral Sclerosis because the 'pathogenic' bacteria can promote the misfolding of proteins.

Many researchers said and agreed, "genetics load the gun, but diet and lifestyle pull the trigger". This is very true indeed! And the message is clear that healthy lifestyles and a Mediterranean diet can help preserve cognitive function and protect memory. Someone may wonder with a question: Is the Mediterranean diet helping the brain, or it is just a marker for an overall healthy lifestyle? I think the answer is both.

EPILOGUE

The curse of Alzheimer's disease is so damning and unrelenting that for every brain it robs and eradicates, one or more victims including caregivers are being punished and painfully affected. Undoubtedly, Alzheimer's is an intrinsically evil disease, affecting everything the patients have, including their memories and dreams.

Spouses, family members and close friends are woefully forced, not only to witness the cruel and painful disappearance of the minds and bodies of their loved ones, but also increasingly to step in and compensate for the lost abilities of the Alzheimer's sufferers. Very few people can appreciate that the caregivers have a thankless job lasting 24 hours a day, seven days a week, and years, fearfully anticipating bad news that can happen at any time.

We must be more aware of and compassionate for the profound, unmet needs of the patients and caregivers. There are many mitigating and beneficial factors and positive strategies that can change the course of the disease, and it is time for all of us to cast a wider net, even though there is no sure-fire way to avoid the disease, and not one drug to cure the illness at this time.

Early detection and diagnosis is crucial to take advantage of the early stages of the disease, which usually progress slowly over a period of 4 to 8 years. This is a relatively large window of opportunity for proactive and appropriate interventions and strategies, which can reduce its symptoms, slow or halt the progression of this dementing illness, and even regress the conditions.

We must not forget that many studies have demonstrated that the more socially and physically active you are, and the more you participate in mentally stimulating activities, the less likely you are to get Alzheimer's disease or dementia.

During the "redemptive period" of the early stages of the disease, the patients are usually mobile and ambulatory without frailty with most of their cognitive abilities unscathed unless there are serious comorbidities; many studies have shown that regular physical activity including walking, a well-balanced diet with adequate nutritional support, a positive lifestyle with social and mental stimulations can expand the brain reserve and give you a chance to resist the scourge of this horrible disease.

At this time, it is believed that there is no cure for Alzheimer's disease and treatment is focused on improving the quality of life, rightly so, by helping victims maintain brain health, managing their behavioral symptoms, and slowing or delaying its progression, and hopefully halting and reversing the course of this harrowing illness with preemptive, preventive strategies and patient-centered, appropriate intervention.

Many barriers still exist in the current health care system for the Alzheimer's patients and caregivers in their protracted, frustrating, grueling and painful struggle. Concerns about misdiagnosis, uncertainty and misgiving about disclosing the diagnosis, limited availability of specialists and the lack of available treatments, all create considerable challenges and anxiety for the patients and families. Undoubtedly, the strain on the current American healthcare infrastructure will exacerbate as our aging population continues to increase. Alzheimer's disease has already become one of the leading causes of death in the U.S.

Public education and awareness of the disease are imperative in order to quell the fear and misunderstanding of this neurodegenerative chronic illness of Alzheimer's. The United Nations projects that by the year 2050, nearly two billion people in the world will be over the age of 60. But the added years also mean that more older people may spend more time in an incapacitated state in the final stage of the life if we don't act now!

I sincerely pray that all Alzheimer's patients will be spared and blessed with "graceful degradation", able to absorb the damages in their brain without dramatic negative effects on their living and functional performances, so that they can continue to live with dignity and quality in their last exit of the earthly journey.

It is such a paradox that by having extended our lives with the medical advances and technologies, we expand and prolong suffering and frailty. There seems to be no end in sight in the collision course at this juncture. Medical science has given us many tools for staying alive, but it does not help us with the art of living and dying. With Alzheimer's disease, the challenge of the caregivers is to free themselves from the grueling and tormenting confines of the illness, and to find a new humanity in the loss on their own terms. In Alzheimer's disease, the caregivers and loving family kind of experience death and watch its progression in their loved ones like in a slow-motion movie of an inevitable tragedy.

At the end of this slow-motion tragic movie, with the eventual passing of their affected beloved family members, the caregivers with the realization that they are not needed anymore; this forsaken, ambiguous moment is often felt like rushing into the void with a powerful deluge of emotions: relief, guilt, regret, anger, emptiness, desolation and doubt. Many will find themselves searching for a higher sense of purpose in life, and hoping to be whole again with their loved ones.

The social impact and burden of Alzheimer's disease is going to be horrendous, stupendous and unfathomable. From the point of the affected individuals, their pain and suffering and losses are profoundly indescribable; from the point of view of the society, there is a haunting and daunting question in the victims' minds that how long their physical and mental disabilities will be and how much of a burden to the society. With heart diseases and cancers, the period of disability, suffering and dependency is usually brief, averaging 3 to 5 years. With Alzheimer's disease, it can go on as long as 20 years.

Alzheimer's disease, yet, continues to intrigue and confound all of us, including researchers. Whether you are poor or rich, famous or anonymous, or the President of the United States, this neurodegenerative disease does not discriminate. It is undoubtedly a very complex disease with many risk factors, some of which you cannot change such as your age and genes. But, we have been demonstrating and seeing more and more promising and convincing evidences that, through healthy lifestyles and diet, you can significantly reduce your risk of Alzheimer's and dementia.

As a summation, you will increase your risk of Alzheimer's disease and dementia if

- You are not getting adequate sleep
- You are not walking or exercising
- You are not eating a Mediterranean diet
- You are not connecting socially
- You are not drinking red wine in moderation
- You are not keeping a normal, healthy weight
- You are not learning new things
- You are not wearing a helmet or a seat belt
- You are not managing your blood pressure to keep it within normal limit
- You are not watching and managing your blood sugar levels
- You are not doing balance and coordination exercises

We, as a nation and a community of this world, must plan proactively and be ready to take on this moral challenge of Alzheimer's disease and to make a sincere commitment to the prevention and intervention of this daunting dementing illness! In our traditional acute-care- and disease-oriented medical system, we often neglect or minimize the human dimensions of long-term medical care for chronic diseases.

MEMORY RE-EDUCATION TECHNIQUES

Memory loss and other changes in cognition are probably among the most common fears for adults as they age, especially the older adults. Although a mild or modest decline in memory and cognitive functions is to be expected in aging, some changes may be indicative of a larger issue, more than "senior moments" or mild cognitive impairment (MCI).

The brain normally has different memory functions:

- Episodic memory – that is, remembering personal events and experiences, but visio-spatial cognition may be more affected by aging than verbal cognition.
- Prospective memory – it is the ability to remember to perform an action or task in the future.
- Procedural memory – this is referring to the acquisition and later performance of cognition and motor skills. This can be very stable if performed and repeated regularly.
- Working memory – it is the ability of holding, coordinating and manipulating information in the mind, with its processing speed gradually decreasing with age.
- Semantic memory – this is the one function of the brain about facts and general knowledge about the world. It remains relatively stable with age, especially if the information is used frequently.

MEMORY RE-EDUCATION TECHNIQUES

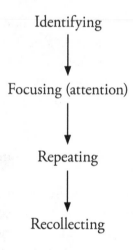

Identifying

↓

Focusing (attention)

↓

Repeating

↓

Recollecting

Identifying:

Here you introduce the person or an object, familiar or new to the patient with Alzheimer's disease. You can explain in simple words who the person is, or what the object is in relation to a specific situation. In this process of identifying, you want to move the object around in front of the patient; movement makes a static image dynamic, creating traction in the brain and making it more memorable.

Focusing (Attention):

The secret of memory is attention. If your attention is not in the right place when something goes by (that you want to remember), you will not remember it no matter how good your memory is. In fact, communication or learning is impossible without paying attention, and attention is at its best with motivation. In this step, you ask the patient to focus on the person or an object to be introduced. There is brain activity when one pays attention, at least one is thinking about it. Perhaps, it may activate or strengthen neural pathways, or form new ones.

It is incontrovertible that focusing or paying attention and memory are intricately related, though the exact mechanisms are not clearly known. Essentially, perception and memory are intricately entwined, and trying to connect different perceptual fragments to stored memories may improve the remembered information. The brain is built to respond to experience; it can change with its malleability and neuroplasticity. This is what learning is in the spectrum of attention-learning-memory.

The power of neuroplasticity of the human brain is unfathomable. When you do something over and over, the brain will grow new connections that undergird what you have learned. This is similar to physical therapy, driving the mechanism of neuroplasticity to restore the functional maps of the brain for the stroke victims.

Repeating:

In this step, you ask the patient to say it after you, and this may be repeated; the auditory and visual pathways are activated in the process of repetition, helping to improve the senses. When the patient is repeating after you, have him or her pointing and gesturing toward the person or object already introduced and identified. When repeating the words and visualizing the object or person introduced, both sides of the brain are working.

Repetition is one of the important and principal ways of remembering things in learning; most of us have spent much of our educational life learning through repetition. How much and how soon the information can be stored and retrieved by the patient is dependent upon the severity of the illness. I recommend the practice of this "Memory Re-education Technique" between the patient and the caregiver or the reminiscence therapist in the early stages of Alzheimer's disease before the symptoms of dementia become overwhelming in the late stages of the disease.

The caregivers and caring family members have nothing to lose in this in-person encounter but everything to gain. Please be reminded that you show the patient something or do something that is simple, just to get into the mind-set of confidence. This technique can be applied to many activities of daily living, for example, teaching your impaired loved one how to put on his or her clothes the correct way.

Cognitive stimulation has been proven by many studies to help impaired individuals remember how to complete activities of daily living; it results in positive changes in brain activities that can be observed and measured by functional MRI scans. With this memory re-education technique for the Alzheimer's patients, synergistic benefits can be realized in collaboration with the cognitive rehabilitation therapy (CRT), which aim to restore cognitive function after a brain injury.

THE CONCEPT OF AN
ALZHEIMER'S VILLAGE

Alzheimer's disease is more common among the Caucasians in the West than people in the East, according to epidemiological statistics. Researchers have been looking at the discrepancy of the prevalence between the West and the East, but the precise mechanisms are not very clear at this time. Perhaps, genetics, lifestyles, diets, socio-cultural structures including family interactions, or all of the above.

With the fast- growing elderly population worldwide, the number of people affected by Alzheimer's disease is expected to reach over 130 million by the year 2050, about one generation from now; in the U.S., the current 5.5 million Alzheimer's patients will be increased to about 15.5 million with the trend continuing. These conservative and realistic projections are stunning and mind-boggling, reaching an epidemic proportion soon, if not already here.

Netherlands has started a model of communal living for residents with Alzheimer's disease in Weesp; this special community is known as Hogeweyk. It is going to "take a village" to provide adequate and optimal care for the elderly Alzheimer's sufferers due to the extended period of time for this disease to run its course, its symptomatic unpredictability, and the vulnerability of the impaired individuals including the needs of the caregivers.

In many long-term care facilities (nursing homes) and hospital wards, the residents/patients with Alzheimer's disease and dementia are likely to retreat themselves in the safety of their chairs or lying in beds. This type of settings and surroundings are absolutely NOT what they need, and will only deteriorate their body and mind, and de-humanize their disease processes. They should be removed from the depressing, grim and compromising facilities and hospital-style wards into home-like settings in a planned community, providing these patients with positive human interactions, trained staff in Alzheimer's care, and beneficial physical and mental activities.

All of us will, inevitably and eventually, face aging, dying and death; it is just a matter of time. But our youth-oriented culture in the West seems to be in denial, fearing to confront these life issues, especially Alzheimer's disease. In the Eastern Culture, most families live in villages or in communities where there are many people living in the same household, having an extended family of two to three generations to help each other. The cultural and social interactions of dependence, independence and inter-dependence are clearly observed among them.

This brings us another human dimension of Alzheimer's disease. When I was a medical student in the 1970s, I I did not hear much about Alzheimer's disease, which was considered. Nowadays, Alzheimer's has become a household name and the mere mention of it is imbued with trepidation and fear. This is understandable because the number of people suffering from Alzheimer's disease has been rising steadily both in the U.S. and across the globe.

We are a tribal species with close ties to the families, up until the second half of the 20th century when individual mobility increasing and spreading. We are witnessing more and more people moving away from their family settings in villages and communities, causing the break-down of the natural order of family care-taking and inter-dependence. Gradually, the elderly members of the families are facing 'abandonment' in the later years of their lives along with the loss of respect and value as heads of the families. Fears of providing for oneself in one's old age sadly created a new dimension of stress in our modern society, which have changed to revolve intensely around remaining young.

It is my belief that Alzheimer's disease, among its multiple causative factors, is also related to the breakdown of the family units and weakening of the family bonds that once extended naturally from birth to death. It is rather notable that this dementing illness has grown in proportion to the changing patterns of modern-day society with the withdrawal of the conscious minds of the elderly family members. This phenomenon or state of giving up and withdrawing sub-consciously from their involvements in the family situations is a form of social resignation, I believe.

The Eastern culture considers the fading of the mind with some degree of dementia a natural aging process, just like the weakening and frailty of the physical body eventually. However, due to the strong spirit and belief in the community and extended family, the older members remain with dignity in the tightly-knit social network. Caregiving for the impaired and debilitated elderly is shared by many more family members and friends than the nuclear families in the West, in general.

In the Eastern traditions, ending one's life at advanced age, even in the face of terminal illness is regarded as interfering with the natural destiny. When the final exit comes on the earthly journey, the sojourner will go ahead and explore the next journey, preparing the way for the younger generations.

In the U.S., there are Alzheimer's long-term care centers with day programs for family and caregivers to rely upon when the needs arise. But this is a far cry from the concept of Alzheimer's Village, a community designed for the special, unique needs and care of the Alzheimer's patients. The concept of the sacred dimension of 'graceful aging' and death with dignity may seem counter-cultural to us in the West at this time. We must contemplate and accept the "gifts of aging", so that we will be ready with open hearts when our time comes, sooner or later.

ADDENDUM

SPIRITUALITY AND FAITH

Taking care of your loved one with Alzheimer's Disease is very challenging, frustrating and grueling, to say the least. Personally witnessing him or her losing themselves, forgetting their friends and family, and toward the end, becoming totally dependent, and disconnected from the world around them. This undoubtedly can cause incredible stress and immeasurable emotional toll on the caregivers in this heart-breaking, long and uncertain journey. Looking at this unrelenting, harrowing and devastating disease from a spiritual perspective may illuminate this protracted process of caring for someone with Alzheimer's.

Until recently, very little attention is paid to the emotional component and the strain that stress can create and become an important factor in many illnesses. Some medications may be effective in treating the different reactions to stress sometimes, but not the core of stress itself. There is a plethora of evidence that negative emotions and stress do impact our health adversely. Even though the traditional medical community has been taking a more cautious approach in reaching the inclusions on this subject, nowadays, the door is widely opened for the holistic approach, including spirituality and faith.

The point of bringing a spiritual perspective into your life is to remind yourself that you are more than just your own physical body, and that there is more to life than the material world. We are actually spiritual beings inhabiting the material/physical forms. I believe, nothing is random in life: the miraculous make-up of the human body, the wonders of nature, the complex and inexplicable creation of birth, and the profound earthly journey from the beginning to the end.

Spirituality and health are inextricably and profoundly linked as more and more studies have found, and this observed in many different cultures of the world. Metaphysically, life lives at the expense of other life. It does not matter whether you are a carnivore, omnivore or a vegetarian, you sustain and perpetuate your physical existence by taking the lives of other organisms.

Just take a brief moment before eating to contemplate and to remember our dependence upon other living things and our need to take other lives in order to sustain and perpetuate life. It should be time to feel gratitude for the foods you are about to eat. The ancient philosophers and thinkers told us that this is the direction in which we all will find comfort, peace and equanimity.

Life is indeed full of changes and vicissitudes; the longer you live, the more changes you will encounter. Changes can be uplifting, challenging and energizing; sometimes they can be disheartening and devastating such as the diagnosis of Alzheimer's Disease or incurable cancer, enough to shake you to your roots. What sustains and bolsters you, and keeps you steady and resilient when it feels as though the earth is shaking and moving beneath your feet? For many people, the answer is their faith. Faith means not only a belief in a Higher Power, but also social connections to others. With Alzheimer's Disease, as with any serious, life-threatening illness, we are essentially powerless in the face of insuperable and uncontrollable event or process; many of us turn to our faith for strength, peace, equanimity and love.

Many people today tend to under-value and doubt faith, assuming that it means believing without any real proof or evidence. Faith, to me, is more than belief; it is not gullibility, and it is not superstition. We must keep an open mind; there is a saying that "absence of evidence is NOT evidence of absence". Faith is very personal, close to you and deep within you. Faith focuses on something hoped for, but has not yet happened. Faith is imbued with gratitude for something positive experienced, which is observable, but not measurable like in a laboratory. In essence, our physical eyes cannot see the realities in the spiritual realm.

It is easier for many people to say that the Universe is created by chance or other plausible theories. With the flow and movements that sustain all forms of life, it is my faith to believe that a Higher Power, or some people call the Supreme Being or God, is in control. Of course, nobody should be persuaded or forced into believing in something that requires faith. I have nothing against skeptics or atheists, or agnostic; it is a personal choice.

As a physician educated in the West and trained to think scientifically for many years, even in the field of clinical medicine, we cannot always find an explanation for all the symptoms patients present, we call the ailment idiopathic, or etiology unknown. When a patient has spontaneous remission of a cancer without reasonable and acceptable explanation, the treating physician is often puzzled and confounded, calling the phenomenon a "fluke", or a stroke of fortune.

When you are a believer in God, you put your faith in God to protect and sustain you through crises and trial, such as the diagnosis of Alzheimer's disease. You will still proactively manage the disease, but you trust that God has a plan for your life and His love will carry you through with assurance and resilience.

Even when death approaches in the final days of Alzheimer's, you will find comfort with your faith, knowing that your God loves you and your suffering loved one, and this is just a passing phase of this earthly journey, liberating you from the body, the mind and the disease. You are able to draw remarkable emotional and physical strength from your faith, which gives you optimism and hope, admittedly powerful tools in survival!

When you have faith, you know that you are never alone in your struggle. Faith is ineffable, and to some, mysterious. The faithfuls don't need science or studies to support their conviction because they don't require them. Spirituality is a rather broad term that includes a sense of connection to some being bigger and higher than oneself. It is a set of personal feelings, or it can be part of organized religion. Spirituality, in actuality, a search for the sacred and divine Power.

There is a lot of overlapping with spirituality and faith (or religion), and the health benefits for the body and mind are essentially the same or very similar.

Spirituality deals with the non-physical parts of you, such as the way you think and feel. It often points to the fundamental human quest for understanding the ultimate truth of human existence. While its concept is personal, private and individual, religion brings together people of similar beliefs and similar spirituality. In fact, spiritual experiences are surprisingly common, even among those who describe themselves as non-religious. These individuals often admit that there are things that cannot be explained or touched, but they believe in the existence of spiritual beings.

Psychoneuroimmunology, a field of medical science that studies how your mind influences your health and how social and psychological factors, such as religion, affect the immune and nervous systems. The impact of faith in the lives of almost 80% of the world's population who are involved in organized religion is enormous and undeniable. Religion is a system of spiritual practices that guide the faithfuls or believers on a spiritual journey deep in the soul and mind. Nevertheless, one can be religious without any formal participation in open religious services; it is your personal relationship with your God. Due to the supportive, interacting relationships, many attend churches, mosques, temples and synagogues.

There is a growing body of evidence in social and psychological science studies that religious people are happier, healthier, and recovering better after traumas than non-religious people. Comparing with the non-religious and non-spiritual individuals, people active in their religion report greater social support, most likely, through the church or other organizational establishment itself, and live longer with a variety of illnesses in general.

Many studies have shown that religious patients, after cardiac surgeries, live longer with longer survival rates probably due to strength, comfort and hope from their faith. Another reason, according to researchers, could be that religious people are more likely to have healthier behaviors and lifestyles with positive outlooks and harmonious family life. On average, religious people suffer less from anxiety and depression than non-religious counterparts, and are less prone to suicide, less likely to smoke, and less likely to abuse drugs or alcohol.

After all, religion is usually not practiced in isolation (except those in contemplative solitude) but within a fellowship of kindred spirits, and share one another's burdens, reach out to those in need and offer assistance when possible, friendship and companionship. Most of the research and social studies have shown that people who attend church regularly live about 7 years longer than those who don't. Dr. David Koenig of Duke University Medical Center, as founder and Director of the Center for the Study of Religion, Spirituality and Health has written more than 35 books and hundreds of articles on how religious beliefs and observance positively influence mental and physical well-being.

He states that "religious attendance produces" positive psychological, social and behavioral consequences. In short, church-goers and religious people usually do not drink or engage in risky businesses.

The power of praying, either for yourself or another person, is indescribable and inexplicable. In our world of modern science, it is controversial because it is difficult to measure or quantify the impact of one's prayers. However, many studies have shown that praying for oneself and intercessory prayers can actually lead to positive results. For example, researchers at Duke University Medical Center found cardiac patients who received stents and prayers recovered better than those with stents only, given very similar background conditions and medical history. In fact, there is more and more convincing research linking prayers with positive health outcomes. Some people demand empirical proof for the power of prayers, and/or the presence of God, and I think, such pursuit is futile. Miracles and the power of prayers may be impossible to verify in a scientific study or measure in a laboratory conclusively and precisely beyond reasonable doubt, but that is exactly and ultimately the point.

In difficult, heart-rending and harrowing situations such as providing care for your loved one afflicted with Alzheimer's disease, it is good and beneficial for anyone to seek a way to cultivate spiritual resilience and serenity. It is time to surrender, it does not mean giving up or resignation, but rather it suggests letting go and trusting your God. It means having faith in the Higher Power beyond your limited self, and the "surrender" will bring you peace, strength and calmness with renewed purpose and meaning, even in the face of tragedy and death.

I would like to close this segment and this book with two quotes, from my perspective of Alzheimer's Disease. The first one from the French priest, philosopher and mystic, Teilhard de Chardin: "In my younger years, I thanked God for this expanding, growing life. In my later years, when I found my physical powers growing less, I thanked God also for what I called the Grace of Diminishment".

The second quote is from the book written by Ram Dass titled "Still Here: Embracing Aging, Changing, and Dying". He said, "Because my memory has been affected, I am no longer bound to past and future in some way, and the relief of this is enormous. For this reason, illness and aging contain the seeds of great opportunity in terms of spiritual growth".

In dying, you are no longer imprisoned by the physical body. The spiritual healing of death will bring you serenity, renewed purposes and direction, from deterioration to transformation!

CPSIA information can be obtained
at www.ICGtesting.com
Printed in the USA
LVHW011131200222
711571LV00003B/45